HOSPITALISTS

A Guide to Building and Sustaining a
Successful Program

HOSPITALISTS

A Guide to Building and Sustaining a Successful Program

Joseph A. Miller

John Nelson

Winthrop F. Whitcomb

ACHE Management Series

12 11 10 09 08   5 4 3 2 1

Library of Congress Cataloging-in-Publication Data

Miller, Joseph A., 1948-
    Hospitalists : a guide to building and sustaining a successful program / Joseph A. Miller, John Nelson, and Winthrop F. Whitcomb.
    p. ; cm.
    Includes bibliographical references and index.
    ISBN-13: 978-1-56793-283-6 (alk. paper)
    1. Hospitalists. 2. Hospitals--Personnel management. I. Nelson, John, 1959- II. Whitcomb, Winthrop F. III. Title.
[DNLM: 1. Hospitalists--organization & administration. 2. Hospitalists--manpower. 3. Personnel Staffing and Scheduling--organization & administration. WX 203 M648h 2007]
RA972.M45 2007
362.11068'3--dc22

                                                              2007036032

The paper used in this publication meets the minimum requirements of American National Standard for Information Sciences—Permanence of Paper for Printed Library Materials, ANSI Z39.48-1984. ∞™

Acquisitions editor: Audrey Kaufman; Project manager: Jane Calayag;
Cover designer: Chris Underdown

Health Administration Press
A division of the Foundation of the
    American College of Healthcare Executives
1 North Franklin Street, Suite 1700
Chicago, IL 60606–3529
(312) 424–2800

Contents

Foreword: The Future Role
of Hospitalists

Since the mid-1990s, when Robert Wachter and Lee Goldman (1996) first coined the term "hospitalist," we have seen the nation's hospitals and health systems open their doors to these "specialists in inpatient medicine." We have also seen publications and academic studies that outline the benefits of implementing hospitalist programs. As the chief executive officer of an integrated delivery system, I can recount firsthand how our hospitalist program, in existence since 1995, has improved patient care in our facilities. Not only have our hospitalists saved the system thousands of days in length of stay and reduced our costs per day, but they have also improved quality of care. In addition, members of our hospitalist groups have emerged as physician liaisons, championing education and training initiatives and serving as a bridge between the medical staff and management. As our experience and this book suggest, hospitalists add value on multiple levels and have embedded a new model of care within the nation's hospitals.

What's next? How will hospitalists continue to improve the comprehensiveness and continuity of healthcare across the patient care continuum? And, perhaps more importantly, how do we get there from here?

While hospital programs are burgeoning, many hospitals and health systems have yet to realize the full value added by hospitalist programs. One role that hospitalists may increasingly assume is that of a change agent. The nature of the hospitalist's work ideally enables him to identify process improvement initiatives and corral physician support. As a result, hospitalists will increasingly serve as administrative partners and leaders of medical staff initiatives to help facilitate organizational change.

In addition to serving as change agents, hospitalists themselves may become the solution to systems that need changing. In many institutions, they are already helping to solve on-call challenges by providing 24/7 on-site coverage and by taking unassigned general medicine or pediatric emergency calls. Hospitalists have also assumed a greater role in caring for patients in the emergency department by managing patients who otherwise would have been admitted by on-call physicians. As more and more physicians decrease the time they spend in the hospital and as more patients are admitted with chronic care needs, the hospitalist will play an integral role in meeting these challenges.

Hospitalists may also become more involved in providing continuity to the delivery of healthcare services. Hospitalists can help resolve the disconnect that exists as a patient moves across the continuum of care. A patient may enter the system through the intensive care unit, followed by a transfer to a medicine unit, and then be discharged to her primary care physician or a nursing home. The reality of ineffective communication and incomplete handoffs may result in poor information exchange that affects the care of the patient. By involving a hospitalist in this process, the coordination of patient care becomes seamless and the chance for medical error decreases.

To expand the current hospitalist model to the clinically diverse and dynamic model of the future, all stakeholders, from management to physicians, must take proactive steps. Part of this process will involve the development of an economic model that accounts for the value that hospitalist programs bring. The more quantifiable these programs become, the easier it will be to prove their value and implement them in capital-strapped facilities. Chapter 4, on return on investment, provides a framework for measuring the costs and benefits of a hospitalist program.

Another part of moving the hospitalist model to the future centers on relationship management. A lack of understanding of the benefits that hospitalists provide and the roles that they assume in hospitals prevents collaboration with other specialties. Lines of communication must be opened and issues of distrust must be resolved to facilitate the relationships among hospitalists, the medical staff, and management. Finally, we must educate the community about the benefits of hospitalists in the delivery of patient care. Chapter 9, on communication, outlines some best practices that hospital leaders should consider for their hospitalist program.

This book offers hospital executives concrete, practical advice on how to build and sustain a well-managed hospitalist program. It covers a wide range of topics—from scheduling to performance reporting—that must be addressed to achieve success with regard to quality of care, throughput, the bottom line, and medical staff satisfaction.

David L. Bernd, FACHE,
chief executive officer, Sentara Healthcare, and
past president, American Hospital Association

REFERENCE

Wachter, R. M., and L. Goldman. 1996. "The Emerging Role of 'Hospitalists' in the American Healthcare System." *New England Journal of Medicine* 335: 514–17.

ADDITIONAL READINGS

American Hospital Association. 2003. *Annual Survey of the American Hospital Association.* Chicago: American Hospital Association.

Olsen, K., and R. Wachter. 2004. "The Word on Medical Mistakes." *Health Leaders Speak Out*. [Online article; retrieved 2/24/07.] www.healthleaders.com/news/feature57663.html.

Preface

Consider the following facts:

- Results from the 2005 *Annual Survey* of the American Hospital Association indicate that more than 16,000 hospitalists were practicing in the United States, a 40 percent growth over a two-year period.
- The same survey indicates that approximately 40 percent of the 4,800 community hospitals in the United States had hospitalist programs; for hospitals with 200 or more beds, the penetration of hospitalists was 70 percent.
- Assuming conservative growth rates, the number of hospitalists reached 20,000 in 2007 and will reach 30,000 in 2010.

With fewer than 1,000 hospitalists—inpatient specialists in the practice of medicine—in 1996, these facts confirm that hospital medicine is "the fastest growing physician specialty in history" (Society of Hospital Medicine 2007). (It took emergency medicine 20 years to reach 20,000 physicians; hospital medicine did it in just more than 10 years.)

Despite these startling statistics, the impact of hospital medicine has not been fully recognized by all segments of the healthcare industry, the press and media, and consumers. Furthermore, given the youth of the hospitalist movement, many if not most hospitalist programs have not reached their full potential.

This book is targeted to hospital executives and hospitalist leaders seeking to improve the performance of their hospital medicine group. It aims to describe and characterize best practices and successful models within the fast-growing hospitalist movement.

The book has two sections:

- *Section I—Hospital Medicine: A Strategic Perspective.* Chapters 1 through 6 look at hospital medicine from a "30,000 foot" perspective. These chapters provide an overview of the hospital medicine specialty, a discussion of the contributions that can be made by hospitalists, a framework for evaluating a return on investment, a high-level summary of dos and don'ts, and a description of an organizational–legal framework that creates incentives for ensuring the success of a hospitalist program.
- *Section II—Hospital Medicine: A Practice Management Perspective.* The remaining chapters focus on the details of implementing and sustaining a successful hospital medicine group. Each chapter examines a subject in detail, describing best practices; identifying relevant tools and techniques; and referencing research, surveys, and the authors' extensive collective experience. The topics are retention and career satisfaction, use of nonphysician staff, communications, staffing, scheduling, night coverage, compensation, the role of the medical director, performance measurement, information systems, billing revenue, and practice management issues for pediatric hospitalist programs.

To further illustrate some of the concepts discussed in the book, we have included examples of various elements germane to a hospitalist program. These tools are presented as appendixes at the end of the book. These appendixes, and other supplemental documents, appear on the publisher's Book Companion website at ache.org/books/Hospitalists.

With regard to the terminology used in the book, a series of terms are used interchangeably to describe a group of doctors working as hospitalists—hospital medicine group, hospital medicine program, hospitalist program, hospitalist group, and hospitalist practice. Also, we have used the term "nocturnist," which is becoming a commonly accepted term for doctors who principally or exclusively work at night.

Hospitals are being challenged with the realities of an aging population, fiscal constraints, and the increased use of technology. Hospitalists can partner with hospital executives to address these challenges.

ACKNOWLEDGMENT

We would like to acknowledge the support of the leaders and staff of our respective organizations—Society of Hospital Medicine, Mercy Medical Center, and Overlake Hospital Medical Center—in making this book possible.

Joseph A. Miller
John Nelson, M.D.
Winthrop F. Whitcomb, M.D.

REFERENCES

American Hospital Association. 2005. *Annual Survey.* Chicago: American Hospital Association.

Society of Hospital Medicine. 2007. "Hospital Medicine Specialty Shows 20 Percent Growth." [Online press release; retrieved 3/14/07.] www.hospitalmedicine.org/AM/Template.cfm?Section=Press_Releases&Template=/CM/ContentDisplay.cfm&ContentID=12507.

SECTION I

HOSPITAL MEDICINE:
A STRATEGIC PERSPECTIVE

CHAPTER 1

Hospitalists: Why the Concept Works[1]

Key Message

A number of innate qualities of the hospitalist model create benefits for hospitals.

Hospital executives, when they are introduced to the concept and potential benefits of a hospitalist, often nod their heads in agreement. There is a compelling logic to creating an inpatient specialist role in the hospital that has the potential to improve performance and provide multidimensional value to a range of stakeholders. Figure 1.1 describes this value equation, answering the questions of how and why hospitalists provide value or, put another way, why the hospitalist model works. The diagram depicts three elements:

- *The characteristics of hospitalists:* These are the attributes that uniquely define this new physician specialty.
- *The expertise of hospitalists:* As they practice hospital medicine, hospitalists have developed a unique combination of knowledge, skills, and relationships.

Figure 1.1. The Hospitalist Value Chain

```
┌─────────────────────────────────────────────────┐
│          Characteristics of Hospitalists          │
│   • Inpatient practice                            │
│   • Consistent in-hospital presence               │
│   • Cohesive physician group                      │
└─────────────────────────────────────────────────┘
                         ↓
┌─────────────────────────────────────────────────┐
│            Expertise of Hospitalists              │
│   • Inpatient clinical knowledge                  │
│   • Inpatient clinical skills                     │
│   • Organizational knowledge and relationships    │
│   • Healthcare industry knowledge                 │
└─────────────────────────────────────────────────┘
                         ↓
┌─────────────────────────────────────────────────┐
│           Value Added by Hospitalists             │
│   • Treating unassigned patients                  │
│   • Leading hospital medical staffs               │
│   • Improving physicians' practices               │
│   • Providing extraordinary availability          │
│   • Improving resource utilization                │
│   • Maximizing throughput and improving patient flow │
│   • Educating through formal/informal learning processes │
│   • Improving patient safety and quality of care  │
└─────────────────────────────────────────────────┘
```

- *The valued added by hospitalists:* Hospitalists affect a wide range of issues that address the patient care, financial, and strategic goals of the hospital.

THE CHARACTERISTICS OF HOSPITALISTS

The first attribute that differentiates hospitalists from other medical specialties describes what hospitalists do. Hospitalists have an inpatient practice. Their day consists of admitting, rounding, managing, discharging, and consulting for hospitalized patients. In the traditional model of inpatient care, office-based physicians treat inpatients for only a fraction of their professional time. Hospitalists develop and hone a skill set based on continuous exposure to acutely ill hospitalized patients.

The second attribute describes where hospitalists practice; they have a consistent in-hospital presence. As a consequence, hospitalists do the same or similar activities and relate to the same people in the same place on a daily basis. Unlike community physicians who practice in multiple settings (office and hospital), hospitalists spend all of their time in one environment.

The third attribute describes how hospitalists are organized. A hospitalist practice is a cohesive physician group, and like any other medical group, the members develop a common organizational identity, a consistent practice philosophy, and a balance of individual and communal goals. However, the characteristics and concerns of a hospitalist group are likely to be different from those of a group of office-based internists, surgeons, oncologists, or psychiatrists.

THE EXPERTISE OF HOSPITALISTS

As inpatient generalists, hospitalists continually treat the most common medical conditions that require hospital admission, thus acquiring exceptional clinical knowledge of the conditions and issues involved in managing patients with multiple comorbidities. In addition, hospitalists are familiar with the clinical tools that support the patient care process.

In addition to clinical knowledge, hospitalists have inpatient clinical skills, which include diagnosis, physical examination, discharge planning, medical chart recording, family meeting coordination and oversight, and the performance of technical procedures.

Through their constant presence in the hospital, hospitalists develop exceptional organizational knowledge and relationships. They are familiar with the way patients move through their hospital and the impact of hospital processes, procedures, rules, regulations, and information systems on that patient flow. They understand how to get things done in their facility and often have well-developed relationships with other hospital-based professionals and hospital departments.

Hospitalists typically are the most knowledgeable inpatient clinicians with regard to a wide range of healthcare industry issues. These include comprehension of hospital quality and patient safety practices, the payer/insurance regulations, state and federal regulations, public health initiatives, recently enacted or pending healthcare legislation, and financial issues facing their hospital.

Another framework for defining the expertise of hospitalists is outlined in a publication of the Society of Hospital Medicine (SHM 2006) entitled *The Core Competencies in Hospital Medicine: A Framework for Curriculum Development*. It defines three dimensions of competencies: clinical conditions, procedures, and healthcare systems. A total of 51 competencies are identified, as shown in Table 1.1.

For each of these 51 competencies, *The Core Competencies* describes what hospitalists should be able to do with regard to four dimensions: knowledge, skills, attitudes, and system organization and improvement. Using these competencies, SHM is seeking to define the hospitalist skill set. At the same time, the American Board of Internal Medicine has decided to certify hospitalists in a "recognition of focused practice" that will provide formal acknowledgment of expertise in hospital medicine.

THE VALUE ADDED BY HOSPITALISTS

Hospitalists provide a unique value to hospitals and other major stakeholders in the healthcare industry. Each of the eight different dimensions of value provided by hospitalists is summarized in the following sections and discussed at length in Chapter 3.

First, hospitalists provide an effective solution to hospitals that are having a difficult time organizing their medical staff to provide general medical care for unassigned patient care.

Table 1.1. Core Competencies in Hospital Medicine

Clinical Conditions	Procedures	Healthcare Systems
• Acute coronary syndrome	• Arthrocentesis	• Care of elderly patients
• Acute renal failure	• Chest radiograph interpretation	• Care of vulnerable populations
• Alcohol and drug withdrawal	• Electrocardiogram interpretation	• Communication
• Asthma	• Emergency procedures	• Diagnostic decision making
• Cardiac arrhythmia	• Lumbar puncture	• Drug safety, pharmacoeconomics, pharmacoepidemiology
• Cellulitis	• Paracentesis	• Equitable allocation of resources
• Chronic obstructive pulmonary disease	• Thoracentesis	• Evidence-based medicine
• Community-acquired pneumonia	• Vascular access	• Hospitalist as consultant
• Congestive heart failure		• Hospitalist as teacher
• Delirium and dementia		• Information management
• Diabetes mellitus		• Leadership
• Gastrointestinal bleeding		• Management practices
• Hospital-acquired pneumonia		• Nutrition and hospitalized patients
• Pain management		• Palliative care
• Perioperative medicine		• Patient education
• Sepsis syndrome		• Patient handoff
• Stroke		• Patient safety
• Urinary tract infection		• Practice-based learning and improvement
• Venous thromboembolism		• Prevention of healthcare-associated infections and antimicrobial resistance
		• Professionalism and medical ethics
		• Quality improvement
		• Risk management
		• Team approach and multidisciplinary care
		• Transitions of care

A second issue of concern for hospitals relates to the fact that many physicians are no longer able or willing to serve on hospital committees or play a medical staff leadership role. Hospitalists have emerged as strong candidates to take on this responsibility in their hospitals.

Third, hospitalists provide value by helping to improve physician practices. Primary care physicians, surgeons, emergency physicians, and specialists can benefit from the unique expertise and services provided by hospitalists.

The round-the-clock, on-site coverage provided by many hospitalist programs can be a significant improvement over traditional physician on-call systems. Thus, a fourth value added by hospitalists relates to the provision of extraordinary coverage (often 24/7 on-site coverage).

The dominant challenge facing American hospitals relates to financial pressures. Published research studies have consistently documented that hospital medicine programs generate resource utilization savings—the fifth value added by hospitalists.

Improved throughput management is a sixth value added by hospitalists. Many hospitals are operating at or close to capacity, creating a crisis of bed availability. Hospitalists are uniquely qualified to address these patient flow issues.

A seventh dimension of the value provided by hospitalists relates to the formal and informal education they provide. In a formal capacity, hospitalists are teachers of clinical and nonclinical inpatient skills to medical students, residents, and fellows. In an informal role, hospitalists impart knowledge to other physicians, healthcare professionals, patients, families, and hospital administrators.

Hospitalists make major contributions to healthcare quality and patient safety—the eighth aspect of value added by this specialty. Hospitalists can reduce medical errors, improve the process of care, and achieve better patient outcomes.

CONCLUSION

Hospital medicine has developed as a specialty with unique characteristics and expertise. Hospitalists have specialized skills, knowledge, and relationships that contribute value to hospitals and other stakeholders, including other physicians, patients, and health plans.

These benefits include and go beyond the delivery of quality patient care to hospital inpatients. The hospital medicine specialty continues to grow at a significant rate because of the broad-based positive impact made by hospitalists.

NOTE

1. Some of the material in this chapter has been adapted from Miller, J. A. 2005. "Introduction from the Editor: How Hospitalists Add Value." The Hospitalist 9 (suppl. 1): 6–7.

REFERENCE

Society of Hospital Medicine (SHM). 2006. *The Core Competencies in Hospital Medicine: A Framework for Curriculum Development*. Philadelphia, PA: Society of Hospital Medicine.

CHAPTER 2

Hospitalist Organizational Models

Key Message

Distinct differences exist among the five major organizational models for hospital medicine groups.

There are five major organizational models for hospital medicine groups, defined by the employer of hospitalists:

1. Hospital or hospital-owned corporation
2. Academic institution
3. Multispecialty/primary care medical group
4. Local hospitalist-only group
5. Multistate hospitalist-only group/management company

Figure 2.1 indicates how the approximately 2,500 hospital medicine groups in the United States are distributed among these five models (SHM 2006). The major characteristics of each of these models are described in the following sections. A comparison of these models across 11 key practice management issues is presented in Appendix A at the end of the book.

Figure 2.1. Distribution of Hospital Medicine Groups by Organizational Model

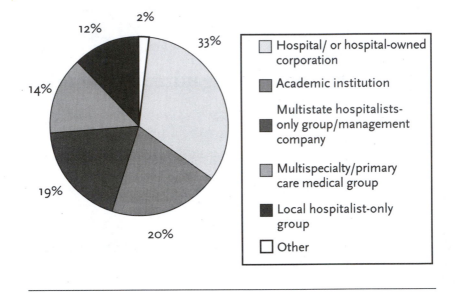

HOSPITALISTS EMPLOYED BY HOSPITALS OR HOSPITAL-OWNED CORPORATIONS

Hospital medicine groups, in which the hospitalists work for a hospital or a hospital-owned corporation, represent approximately 33 percent of the programs in the United States. This type of program is initiated by the hospital to address specific issues and concerns of the hospital (e.g., to provide care to unassigned patients). Often, the hospitalist medical director reports to the vice president of medical affairs or the chief medical officer. Sometimes, the hospitalist medical director reports to a lay administrator (e.g., vice president or director of physician services).

This organizational structure creates a strong alignment between the hospitalists and the hospital in terms of the vision and goals of the hospital medicine group. However, depending on the perspectives of the hospital leadership team, their vision and goals for hospitalists can differ substantially. For some hospitals, the hospitalist role is viewed as simply treating hospitalized medical patients. At other hospitals, the leaders may view hospitalists as a strategic asset that addresses critical issues such as pay for performance, nurse satisfaction, and throughput.

A potential weakness in the hospital-based model is that hospitalists may have an "employee mentality." They may not be as productive or entrepreneurial as physicians who work in a private practice model. Incentive-based compensation can be implemented to create more of an "ownership mentality" for hospitalists.

Because the hospital owns and subsidizes the hospitalist practice, the challenge of quantifying the value provided by hospitalists is especially critical. (See Chapter 4 for a discussion on how to do a return-on-investment analysis.)

HOSPITALISTS EMPLOYED BY ACADEMIC INSTITUTIONS

In this model of hospital medicine group, hospitalists work for an academic medical center or its affiliated medical school. These organizations provide funding to cover the financial deficit of the hospitalist program. Academic hospital medicine groups represent approximately 20 percent of all hospitalist programs in the United States. In this model, the hospitalist medical director typically reports within the division of general internal medicine (for an adult medicine hospitalist program) or the division of pediatrics (for a pediatric hospitalist program). SHM (2006) survey data indicate that pediatric hospitalists are much more likely to work for an academic model than for other hospitalist organization models.

Significant parallels can be seen between the academic model and the hospital-based model previously described—that is, the hospitalists work for large institutional-based employers. However, academic institutions present some unique issues that must be addressed by hospitalists. Specifically, the reduction in resident work hours mandated by the Accreditation Council for Graduate Medical Education has dictated an expanded role for academic hospitalists. Also, the responsibilities of academic hospitalists often include conducting research and being a clinician educator. As such, an academic hospitalist often does not work as many clinical hours as hospitalists who work in other organizational models.

Academic hospitalists are more likely to be paid on the basis of salary (i.e., with no incentive compensation) and, on average, receive less compensation than hospitalists working for other organizational models. They are also more likely to have off-site night-call arrangements, because house staff are usually available as on-site providers in the hospital.

HOSPITALISTS EMPLOYED BY MULTISPECIALTY/PRIMARY CARE MEDICAL GROUPS

Many multispecialty and primary care medical groups have decided to implement hospitalist services in their practice. For adult medicine (and/or for pediatrics), they decide that a separate group of physicians should be responsible for inpatient care (while the primary care physicians maintain an office-only practice). This model represents 14 percent of all hospitalist programs in the United States.

This model differs significantly from those in which hospitalists are employees of institutions (hospitals and/or medical schools) in that the hospitalists are aligned with the vision and goals of the multispecialty/primary care medical group. Because these medical groups are more likely to contract with health plans on a risk/capitation basis, positive performance under those contracts can often influence the hospitalist's practice. Also, it is likely that the hospitalists will have a clear sense of the healthcare providers preferred by the medical group for referrals (e.g., specialists, extended care facilities).

Under this model, primary care physicians and the hospitalists are partners in the same medical group. This arrangement should simplify and improve handoffs and communication. The primary care physician should be more likely to explain the hospitalist model to a patient being admitted than if the primary care physician was referring to a hospitalist who was not part of the medical group. The medical group may have communication capabilities (e.g., common phone system and e-mail) and systems (e.g., electronic medical record) that facilitate communication between the hospitalist and the primary care physician.

Because the hospitalists are part of a private physician practice, typically they bring an ownership mentality to their work. According to SHM (2006) survey data, hospitalists who work for multispecialty/primary care medical groups have the highest median salary ($178,000) among the five organizational models of hospital medicine groups.

HOSPITALISTS EMPLOYED BY LOCAL HOSPITALIST-ONLY GROUPS

Local hospitalist-only groups represent 12 percent of all hospital medicine groups in the United States. This is a pure private practice model for hospitalists. Hospitalists in a local community establish their own medical group focusing solely on inpatient medicine. By definition, this hospitalist organizational model is more entrepreneurial and market driven.

Under this approach, hospitalists must focus on their customers; they acknowledge the need to deliver and document the service they provide. There are two categories of customers for local hospitalist-only groups:

- Hospitalists seek to contract with hospitals to provide a defined set of services (e.g., care for unassigned patients) for a fee. Rather than implement a hospital-employed model,

hospitals can turn to a local hospitalist-only group to outsource the hospitalist function.
- A second customer group for these hospitalists is composed of community primary care physicians. Hospitalists market to these physicians to get them to refer patients for inpatient services.

Local hospitalist-only groups clearly have an ownership mentality. Their productivity and billing directly affect their pocketbooks. Also, these groups are willing to invest in approaches that are found to be cost effective (e.g., nonphysicians, administrative staff support, information systems).

HOSPITALISTS EMPLOYED BY MULTISTATE HOSPITALIST-ONLY GROUPS/MANAGEMENT COMPANIES

As the hospitalist movement has grown, a number of organizations have built national or multiregional companies offering hospitalist services. Some of these organizations started with a sole focus on hospital medicine, while others have developed as a separate business line in companies that offer other physician outsourcing services (e.g., emergency medicine). The business models vary by organization (e.g., how they define and price their services). This hospitalist model represents 19 percent of the hospital medicine groups in the United States. The five largest multistate hospitalist-only groups and/or management companies are listed in Table 2.1.

As in local hospitalist-only groups, this model of hospital medicine group is entrepreneurial and market driven, with a strong focus on expansion and customer service. Typically, a major focus is placed on physician recruitment and retention as the organization builds additional staffing capacity to support new clients in multiple locations.

Table 2.1. The Largest Multistate Hospitalist-Only Groups/Management Companies

Company	Number of Full-Time Hospitalists	Year Started Hospitalist Services
Cogent	130	1997
EmCare	240	1993
IPC—The Hospitalist Co.	500	1995
PrimeDoc	110	1997
TeamHealth	400+	1993

Source: Jerrard (2007).

These national hospitalist organizations typically invest in infrastructure, with centralized billing services, training, information systems, and support staff. The multistate hospitalist-only groups/management companies build a formal, replicable practice model for hospitalists. They have much "deeper" organizations than the other hospital medicine group models, with senior management, sales/marketing staff, physician leaders, and operations departments selling, building, and supporting multiple hospitalist programs in more than one location. In contracts with multistate hospitalist-only groups/management companies, hospitals must expect to pay a fee that covers the investment in this infrastructure and a reasonable profit margin.

CONCLUSION

The five major models of hospitalist programs are (1) hospital owned, (2) academic based, (3) multispecialty/primary care medical group, (4) local hospitalist-only group, and (5) multistate hospitalist-only group/management company. Each of the models has a unique set of drivers that affect the program's structure and the motivations of hospitalists in the program.

REFERENCES

Jerrard, J. 2007. "Big Kahunas: A Look at Six of Today's Largest Hospital Medicine Organizations and What Makes Them Tick." *The Hospitalist* 11 (2): 31.

Society of Hospital Medicine (SHM). 2006. *2005–2006 SHM Survey: State of the Hospital Medicine Movement.* Philadelphia, PA: Society of Hospital Medicine.

CHAPTER 3

How Hospitalists Add Value

Key Message

Hospitalists provide value to patients, the hospital, other physicians, nurses, other health professionals, health plans, the community, and trainees.

As described in Chapter 1, hospitalists provide benefits that can be classified into eight dimensions:

1. Treating unassigned patients
2. Leading hospital medical staffs
3. Improving physicians' practices
4. Providing extraordinary availability
5. Improving resource utilization
6. Maximizing throughput and improving patient flow
7. Educating through formal and informal learning processes
8. Improving patient safety and quality of care

This chapter provides a more in-depth discussion of how hospitalists provide these benefits.

BENEFIT 1: TREATING UNASSIGNED PATIENTS[1]

Key Message

Hospitalists provide a solution to the problem of admissions for unassigned general medicine and pediatric patients.

Hospital executives may recall the 1970s and 1980s, when indigent patients experienced problems at hospital emergency departments (EDs) around the country. They were refused care and shuttled to other facilities for services. To protect patients against these types of abuses, Congress passed the Emergency Medical Treatment and Labor Act (EMTALA) in 1986 as part of the Consolidated Omnibus Budget Reconciliation Act.

EMTALA mandates that all patients presenting to the ED—regardless of insurance status—receive a medical screening examination and be medically stable prior to transfer to another facility. If a hospital has the facilities to treat the emergency, the patient cannot be transferred to another ED. To address these requirements, every hospital must have physicians on call to assist emergency physicians in assessing and treating unassigned patients. By the late 1990s, as EMTALA requirements took hold, inadequate on-call physician coverage reached crisis proportions and became a front-page issue (Appleby 1999; Taylor 1999; Foubister 1999; Winston and the Advisory Board 2000).

Why are physicians unavailable to provide on-call treatment of unassigned patients in the ED and after admission? Hospital leaders have identified three major reasons for this problem. First, at a minimum, on-call treatment of unassigned patients creates an inconvenience for physicians, taking away from their personal time; further, it can reduce the number of available hours they have to spend with their office-based patients. Second, there are financial disincentives to on-call coverage. Often, unassigned patients presenting in the ED are uninsured or underinsured. On-call physicians frequently do not receive adequate compensation for the task of treating these patients. Finally, on-call duty can bring bureaucratic hassles and/or legal liability for physicians. Dealing with state Medicaid agencies may require addressing administrative requirements, completing paperwork, and paying penalties for not following the rules.

Over the past five to ten years, an increasing number of hospital leaders have employed hospitalists to address the crisis of on-call physician coverage. Although issues related to the availability of on-call specialists and surgeons remain, hospitals that have implemented hospital medicine programs are able to make available hospitalists to triage, admit, and treat unassigned general medicine and pediatric patients.

Those members of a hospital medical staff who are frustrated with their responsibilities to be on call are often the driving force for the creation of a hospital medicine program. Having hospitalists at their institution may mean that primary care doctors do not have to assume the undesirable responsibilities of participating in an on-call schedule. Furthermore, because hospitalists typically do not have an office practice, community physicians still have the opportunity to care for the unassigned patients once they are discharged, thereby building their practice. Hospitals can refer unassigned patients discharged by hospitalists according to an equitable schedule approved by the medical staff. Often, the schedule used to identify which primary care doctor admitted an unassigned patient prior to the arrival of hospitalists is simply converted to the schedule used to identify which doctor is to provide the patient's post-discharge follow-up. By addressing issues related to on-call physician coverage, a hospital can improve medical staff relations.

Often, unassigned patients have significant discharge planning and placement problems, especially those who are uninsured. While these issues can be daunting to office-based physicians, hospitalists usually have a more comprehensive knowledge of the resources of the hospital and closer relationships to the hospital's discharge planning staff to help solve these placement and postdischarge care issues.

Hospital leaders often prefer having hospitalists treat their unassigned patients because they are physicians who understand their institution's objectives, concerns, policies, and procedures. Because they are a relatively small, cohesive group within the institution, hospitalists are usually familiar with the hospital's practice guidelines, medical records documentation requirements, computerized physician order entry (CPOE) systems, quality initiatives, and utilization management requirements.

Conclusion

Given the current economic environment, the issue of treating unassigned and uninsured patients will not soon diminish. Demand is likely to increase with the nationwide growth of the number of uninsured patients. Physician resistance to on-call coverage and the rise of malpractice premiums will continue to create more pressure for hospitals to find solutions to this crisis.

BENEFIT 2: LEADING HOSPITAL MEDICAL STAFFS[2]

Key Message

To address the need for physician leaders, hospital administrators are increasingly looking to hospitalists to address critical strategic and operational challenges.

Hospital leaders recognize the vital role of physicians in addressing a range of critical challenges. These issues include pressures on the bottom line; staffing shortages and dissatisfaction; questions about quality and patient safety; constantly changing technologies; employer and consumer demands for performance metrics; capacity constraints; and increased competition from independent, niche providers of clinical services.

Executives are facing the fact that many physicians are no longer able or willing to serve on hospital committees or to play a leadership role for the medical staff. As a result of the pressures of lost income, managed care requirements, on-call responsibilities, and competition for patients as well as lifestyle concerns, many physicians are reluctant to perform volunteer work that hospitals used to take for granted. McGowan (2004) reports the results of a survey of chief executive officers and physician leaders at 55 hospitals in the Northeast conducted by Mitretek Systems, a healthcare consulting firm, noting that "volunteerism is dead." Physicians expect to be paid for time spent on hospital business; 64 percent of the respondents said their hospital compensates physicians to serve as officers or department heads.

It is increasingly likely that doctors on the hospital's "home team"—hospitalists, intensivists, and ED physicians—will assume more prominent positions on hospital committees.[3] Hospitalists have emerged as strong candidates for providing medical staff leadership for the following reasons:

- Hospitalists spend the majority of their time in the inpatient environment, making them familiar with hospital systems, policies, services, departments, and staff.
- Hospitalists are inpatient experts who possess clinical credibility when addressing key issues regarding the inpatient environment.
- Many hospitalists are hospital employees who understand the trade-offs involved in balancing the needs of the institution with those of the medical staff. Even hospitalists who are not employed by the hospital have an intimate knowledge of the issues that the hospital is facing and are invested in finding solutions to these problems.

Figure 3.1 describes a range of roles that a hospitalist could assume and a range of topics that a hospitalist could address in providing medical staff leadership in a hospital.

Figure 3.1. How Hospitalists Provide Physician Leadership

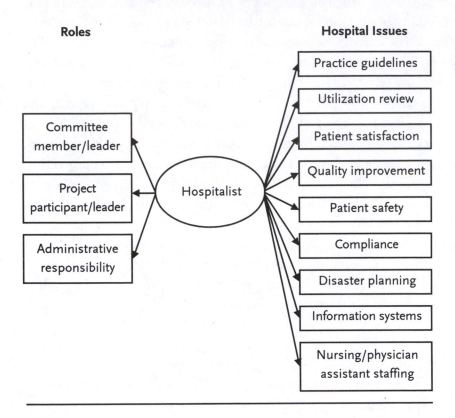

The left side of Figure 3.1 describes three leadership roles that a hospitalist might play in the hospital. First, a hospitalist can volunteer to participate on a hospital committee, either as a member of the committee or as its chairperson. Second, a hospitalist can volunteer to work on a hospital project, either in a staff/expert role or in the role of project leader. Third, a hospitalist can assume an administrative role in the hospital, directing a service or program.

Whether it is through a committee, a project, or direct administrative responsibility, a hospitalist has the knowledge and expertise to become involved in a wide range of hospital issues. As shown on the right side of Figure 3.1, these issues include the following:

- *Practice guidelines.* Many hospitals have adopted practice guidelines as a tool for improving the quality and efficiency of care. When properly developed, guidelines can improve patient safety, facilitate the adoption of best practices, and reduce hospital costs. Hospitalists can be asked to participate in all aspects of guideline development, including research, authorship, implementation, outcome measurement, and ongoing revision and educational efforts.
- *Utilization review.* Hospitals or medical groups routinely arrange for physicians to perform utilization review or improve the utilization review process. A hospitalist can (1) facilitate the discharge process for individual patients, thereby reducing length of stay and hospital costs, and (2) globally improve throughput by identifying and addressing system problems that create inefficiencies in the patient care or discharge process (e.g., paperwork or dictations not completed on time, poor communication across healthcare team disciplines, administrative deficiencies that delay therapies).
- *Patient satisfaction.* Hospitals are increasingly being asked to capture and disseminate performance metrics so that employers and consumers can make informed decisions about their provider of choice. Patient satisfaction is a key measure of a hospital's performance. Hospitalists can become engaged in efforts to review patient satisfaction survey results, identify problems, and propose or implement solutions.
- *Quality improvement.* Many hospitals look to hospitalists to become involved in or lead the hospital's quality improvement (QI) efforts. Specific activities may include championing individual QI projects, working with QI staff to develop and analyze outcomes data, and educating colleagues regarding new projects and protocols.
- *Patient safety.* Preventing harmful errors from occurring in the inpatient environment has become a major priority for hospitals across the United States. Identifying the causes of these errors and developing methods of error prevention require

detailed investigations and analyses of the diagnostic and/or treatment process. Increasingly, hospitalists are being asked to provide leadership to patient safety initiatives.

- *Compliance.* Hospitals must comply with many federal, state, and local rules and regulations. For example, a great deal of coordination and planning is needed to meet the requirements of the Joint Commission, the Health Insurance Portability and Accountability Act of 1996, and the Accreditation Council for Graduate Medical Education (ACGME). In some hospitals, hospitalists assume leadership roles in these compliance efforts.
- *Disaster planning.* Hospitals need to demonstrate the ability to respond to a range of potential crises, including those related to bioterrorism, industrial accidents, and natural disasters (e.g., hurricanes, tornados, earthquakes). In light of their knowledge of patient flow, hospitalists can be asked to work with emergency physicians to do disaster planning for the hospital and the local region.
- *Information systems.* Several organizations (e.g., the Institute of Medicine, the Leapfrog Group, the eHealth Initiative, the Markle Foundation, and the federal Office of the National Coordinator for Health Information Technology) have issued reports identifying information technology as a critical tool for improving healthcare quality. Hospitals are being encouraged and motivated to implement electronic health records and CPOE systems. Implementing these systems requires significant clinical input. Many hospitals have asked hospitalists to champion and lead the implementation process of new information systems.
- *Nursing/physician assistant staffing.* A wide range of roles exists for nurses and physician assistants in the inpatient setting. Every institution needs to find a staffing model that is efficient, is effective, and results in provider satisfaction. Hospitalists are considered leaders of the inpatient medical team and can be asked to help design and evaluate staffing models.

A survey conducted by the Society of Hospital Medicine (SHM 2006a) documents the medical staff leadership roles of hospitalists. On average, hospitalists spend 10 percent to 12 percent of their time on nonclinical activities. Table 3.1 indicates the proportion of the almost 400 hospitalist practices surveyed that are performing specified nonclinical activities.

Conclusion

Hospital administrators need physician leaders to address critical strategic and operational issues. Given their position as inpatient experts, hospitalists are a logical choice to play this role. In the years ahead, it is likely that hospitalists will assume an increasingly

Table 3.1. Nonclinical Responsibilities of Hospitalists

Activity	Percentage of Groups
Committee participation	92
Quality improvement	86
Practice guidelines	72
Pharmacy/therapeutics committee	64
Utilization review	59
CPOE/information systems	54
Teaching—house staff	51
Teaching—non-MDs	36
Recruit/retain MDs	31
Community service	28
Disaster response planning	25
Research	21

Source: SHM (2006a).

important leadership role within community hospitals and academic medical centers in the United States.

BENEFIT 3: IMPROVING PHYSICIANS' PRACTICES[4]

Primary care physicians, surgeons, specialists, and emergency physicians rely on hospitalists to improve their practices.

In a national study published in 2006, researchers asked hospital leaders to rate more than 60 alignment strategies that affect hospital–medical-staff relations. "Employ hospitalists" was the second highest rated alignment strategy, after "employ intensivists," with 74 percent of the survey respondents rating it a 5 or 6 (with 6 being "very positive") (McGowan 2006). In the following sections, we address how hospitalists improve physician practices for primary care physicians (PCPs), surgeons/specialists, and emergency physicians.

Hospitalists and Primary Care Physicians

Consider the following scenarios:

- When an internist in Iowa was called to see one of his patients in the hospital, he faced a 50-minute round trip plus additional time to find a parking place and catch an elevator. In the time it took for him to see the patient in the hospital, he could have treated five patients in the office (Jackson 2001).
- A Florida osteopath estimated that doctors in his practice were spending 30 percent of their time at the hospital caring for only 5 percent of their patients (Massey 2004).

With an eye toward enhancing their office practices, increasing income, offering patients efficient and effective inpatient treatment, and enjoying a more normal lifestyle, both of these physicians in these two scenarios pursued a growing trend in the healthcare industry: they turned to hospitalists.

Some PCPs do have reservations regarding the involvement of hospitalists in the care of their patients. One concern is the potential reduction in income. According to one estimate, PCPs may incur an average annual decrease in income of $25,000 by forgoing hospital rounds. However, studies indicate that PCPs have the potential to earn as much as $50,000 more by spending time in the office instead of seeing inpatients (Landro 2004).

PCPs have other concerns with the hospitalist model. They worry that they might lose skill and prestige by giving up inpatient visits. Some PCPs might express concerns about continuity of care. These concerns are valid and warrant consideration. However, a well-run hospitalist program will keep communication lines open between hospitalists and PCPs so that patients receive optimal care as both inpatients and outpatients.

Hospitalists and Surgeons/Specialists

Hospitalists have both the expertise and the availability to complement the role of the surgeon in caring for surgical patients. As patient care becomes more complex in general, surgeons are increasingly inclined to engage hospitalists as consultants in the care of their patients. Surgeons may feel that they have insufficient knowledge for managing complex medical problems perioperatively. They may be most comfortable in the operating room (OR) or providing care directly related to the procedure being performed. Also, at times surgeons are unavailable because of OR responsibilities for important pre- and postoperative medical problems. To address these issues, hospitalists have a growing role as consultants to surgeons. In other cases, surgical comanagement programs have emerged, where the surgeon provides focused surgical care while the hospitalist provides overall medical care for patients.

While more research is needed to fully assess the impact of hospitalist–surgeon comanagement, a 2004 Mayo Clinic study of 526 patients showed a modest benefit of this approach in patients having hip and knee surgery. The findings revealed that more patients under hospitalist–orthopedist comanagement were discharged with no complications than those managed by traditional orthopedic surgical teams (61.6 percent versus 48.8 percent). Although no differences were found in major complications between the two groups, 30.2 percent of patients comanaged by hospitalists experienced minor complications, while 44.3 percent of patients managed by traditional orthopedic surgical teams had similar difficulties. These differences were statistically significant. The study also noted that when surveyed, most orthopedic surgeons and nurses preferred the hospitalist–orthopedist comanagement model (Huddleston et al. 2004).

Hospitalists and Emergency Physicians

Hospitalists can positively affect the ED in the following ways:

- *Extraordinary availability.* Emergency physicians appreciate that hospitalists are typically more available than office-based primary care doctors. Hospitalists are often able to visit the patient in the ED personally in a timely way, thereby avoiding the practice of the PCP admitting the patient by phone after speaking briefly with the emergency physician.
- *Improved throughput.* In addition to their availability, hospitalists know how to get things done in the hospital. They can expedite care in the ED and the observation unit,

resulting in fewer backlogs and more efficient patient care. However, one potential downside of the hospitalist model is that delays may occur in admitting patients from the ED when multiple patients require admission at the same time. This bottleneck might not have existed in the pre-hospitalist era, as multiple PCPs could have admitted the patients (either in person or by phone). Hospitalist programs will need to develop creative strategies for these crunch periods.

- *Consistent and reliable care.* Hospitalists are more likely to embrace clinical pathways for the most common clinical diagnoses. This reduces variability in practice patterns and improves outcomes.
- *Better teaching.* In teaching hospitals, residents benefit from the presence of hospitalists. They have the continuous supervision of experienced practitioners who can answer questions and teach on an ongoing basis.

Research Studies

A number of research studies (Table 3.2) support the thesis that hospitalists can effectively and efficiently enhance physician practices.

Conclusion

As hospital medicine programs become increasingly prevalent and accepted, more and more physicians are seeing the value in their presence. Implementing a hospital medicine program has become a major strategy for hospital executives seeking to improve medical staff relations. Table 3.3 summarizes the benefits to PCPs, surgeons and other specialists, and emergency physicians.

Table 3.2. Research Results: Physician Perceptions of Hospitalists

Study	Findings
Internists' perception of hospitalist services after implementation (Auerbach et al. 2003)	• More physicians agreed that "caring for inpatients is an inefficient use of my time" ($p < .001$) • More physicians agreed that "use of a hospitalist service improves quality of care" ($p = .002$) • More physicians disagreed that "use of a hospitalist service diminishes physician career satisfaction" ($p < .001$) • More physicians disagreed that "use of a hospitalist service adversely affects the physician–patient relationship" ($p < .001$)
Physician attitudes toward hospitalist model of care and the prevalence of such programs (Auerbach et al. 2000)	• 51% of respondents believed patients would get better care from hospitalists • 47% of respondents thought patients would get more cost-effective care in a hospitalist system
Evaluation of an inpatient physician system for all patients of an HMO admitted to the general medicine service of an urban teaching hospital (Halpert et al. 2000)	• 90% of PCPs indicated satisfaction and would recommend a similar program to other primary care groups • Medical house staff noted an increase in satisfaction regarding their educational experience with hospitalists
How PCPs perceive hospitalists (Fernandez et al. 2000)	• 41% of PCPs perceived hospitalists increased the overall quality of care • 69% reported that hospitalists did not affect their income • 53% believed hospitalists decreased their workload • 50% believed hospitalists increased practice satisfaction

HMO: health maintenance organization; PCP: primary care physician

Table 3.3. How Hospitalists Provide Benefits to Other Physicians

Physician Group	Benefit
Primary care physicians	• Enable physicians to spend more time with office patients • Allow physicians to potentially generate more revenue • Provide more opportunity for family/personal time • Potentially decrease medical-malpractice insurance premiums • Offer flexibility in scheduling • Act as referral source for new patients • Relieve PCPs from the burden of on-call responsibilities, including unassigned general medicine/pediatric ED calls
Surgeons and other specialists	• Perform preprocedural risk assessments, thus avoiding surgical delays • Allow surgeons and specialists to focus on procedural work by addressing routine medical issues • Coordinate care management with a global patient view • Ensure space and availability for elective surgical cases by facilitating throughput • Act as a liaison between the PCP and the surgeon to ensure optimal patient care • Provide temporary or limited ICU coverage, if needed
Emergency physicians	• Facilitate throughput • Provide timely consultations • Reduce ED backlogs • Coordinate care in the observation unit

PCP: primary care physician; ED: emergency department; ICU: intensive care unit

BENEFIT 4: PROVIDING EXTRAORDINARY AVAILABILITY[5]

Key Message

Hospitalist programs with on-site night coverage can contribute to improvements in hospital efficiency, quality, and nurse retention.

Hospitals have traditionally used physician on-call systems and/or the availability of house staff to provide overnight coverage. These systems are not always effective or efficient for patients, physicians, nursing staff, and other hospital departments, as delay of care may jeopardize patient safety. Further, nurses and house staff become frustrated in trying unsuccessfully to locate on-call physicians in a timely fashion in the case of a medical emergency. And the ED may experience a backlog of patients waiting for admission until the doctor arrives in the morning, creating bottlenecks for other hospital departments.

Many hospital leaders have discovered that hospitalists can alleviate these issues and add direct value to a healthcare facility through the implementation of 24/7 coverage. As shown in Table 3.4, 51 percent of hospitalist programs provide on-site, 24/7 coverage, and another 41 percent provide on-call night coverage.

Table 3.4. Night Coverage Arrangements Provided by Hospitalists

Night Coverage Arrangement	Percentage of Hospitalist Programs
On-site hospitalist	51
On-call hospitalist from home	41
No night coverage arrangement	8

Source: SHM (2006a).

Efficiency, quality of care, and nurse retention are major concerns for hospital administrators. An on-site, round-the-clock hospitalist program can address these issues. Consider the following:

- If an on-site physician is not available, the emergency physician will call the PCP and then prepare "bridging orders"—temporary instructions until the morning, when the patient can be seen, formally evaluated, and admitted by his doctor. The absence of lag time between an emergent situation and the on-site presence of a hospitalist might mean the difference between short-term treatment and rapid discharge and a lengthy hospital stay. Healthcare facilities with on-site 24/7 hospital medicine programs operate in "real time" and can evaluate and admit the patient immediately, potentially reducing the length of stay (LOS) and cost per stay and positively affecting the hospital's bottom line.
- If an on-site, 24/7 hospitalist program is in place, hospitalists can provide consultations for surgical and medical cases on the inpatient unit, regardless of the hour. Sudden changes in patient condition, such as fever, chest pain, hypotension, and mental status, can be addressed immediately, thereby improving quality of care. Traditionally, these problems might be managed over the phone at the discretion of the covering physician without direct patient evaluation.
- The advent of 24/7 hospitalists on-site can provide one way to address issues related to nurse dissatisfaction. The round-the-clock presence of a hospitalist benefits the nursing staff by providing support and relieving them of the burden of making decisions that are more aptly handled by physicians. The support of a physician late at night is especially important given that newer, inexperienced nurses are often assigned to these shifts.

Conclusion

Physician lifestyle, quality of care, and patient safety are the primary reasons that on-site 24/7 hospitalist programs are implemented. While limited research has been conducted on the topic, patient care is most likely improved with round-the-clock medical attention provided in person by doctors who expect to be working, instead of care provided by a doctor who is home trying to sleep, as occurs in the traditional model of hospital care. Other benefits may include reduced LOS, improved throughput, and increased nurse satisfaction.

In this era of increased scrutiny of the healthcare field, expectations are growing that a physician will be available in the hospital around the clock to attend to patients. The use of hospitalists on-site on a 24/7 basis may alleviate the pressures being applied to hospitals and, over the short-term at least, provide a strategic advantage that appeals to a hospital's patient community.

BENEFIT 5: IMPROVING RESOURCE UTILIZATION[6]

Key Message

Extensive evidence indicates that hospitalists can generate a measurable reduction in cost and length of stay.

Multiple studies demonstrate the positive effects that hospitalist programs have on resource utilization. Observational, retrospective, and prospective data analyses have been conducted at community-based hospitals as well as at academic medical institutions. Findings consistently indicate that hospitalist programs result in resource savings. The studies referenced in Table 3.5 summarize research evaluating hospitalist programs and their effects on resource utilization.

Table 3.5. Research Results: Hospitalist Impact on Resource Utilization

Description	LOS Savings	Cost Savings	Other Results
Retrospective cohort analysis comparing initial and long-term hospital utilization of hospitalists and general internists at an urban community hospital (Everett et al. 2004)	Reduction of 16.1%	Reduction of 8.3%	Equivalent mortality and 30-day readmission rates
Prospective, quasi-experimental observational study at an academic teaching hospital staffed by hospitalists and non-hospitalist physicians (Kaboli, Barnett, and Rosenthal 2004)	5.5 vs. 6.5 days ($p = .009$)	Reduction of $917 ($p = .08$)	Similar rates of in-hospital mortality and 30-day readmissions
Evaluation of hospitalist program impact on throughput and other measures over a six-week period at an academic medical center (Gregory, Baigelman, and Wilson 2003)	2.19 vs. 3.45 days ($p < .001$)	$1,775 vs. $2,332 ($p < .001$)	• No differences in 30-day readmission rates • Incremental throughput of 266 patients, adding $1.3 million in profitability
Meta study summarizing previous hospitalist research (Wachter and Goldman 2002)	Average decrease of 16.6%	Average decrease of 13.4%	Equivalent results in quality and patient satisfaction
Evaluation of a hospitalist service with a nurse discharge planner compared to generalist-attended and specialist-attended services (Palmer et al. 2001)	• 4.4 vs. 5.2 (generalists) • 4.4 vs. 6.0 (specialists) ($p < .0001$ for both)	• $4,289 vs. $4,850 (generalists) ($p = .11$) • $4,289 vs. $6,066 (specialists) ($p < .0001$)	• Reduced mortality • Equivalent satisfaction and readmission rates

Why the Hospitalist Is Effective

How do hospitalists reduce LOS and cost per stay? Here are several factors that likely contribute to those performance improvements.

- Because hospitalists are physically on-site, they are better able to react to condition changes and requests for consultations in a timely manner.
- Being intimately familiar with the hospital's systems of care, hospitalists know who to call and how to utilize the services of social workers and other staff when arranging for postdischarge care.
- Hospitalists have a high volume of experience in caring for hospitalized patients. They will see more patients with any given diagnosis than a PCP.
- Hospitalists work as a team, collaborating with emergency physicians, specialists, nurses, social workers, and other hospital-based providers. This cooperative relationship often enables the efficient use of human resources in patient care.
- A consistent on-site presence allows a rapid response to patient conditions and problems. Continuous and close monitoring of patients allows for timely adjustments in their care and timely transfers between care settings (e.g., intensive care unit to floor care), which likely reduces LOS and resources consumed.
- Because the care of many patients is provided by a relatively small number of hospitalists (compared to the many PCPs who would have provided the care previously), variation in care is reduced and compliance with local or national practice guidelines often increases.
- With effective scheduling, hospitalists can improve inpatient continuity of care compared with care provided by office-based doctors. A study at a community teaching hospital examined cases managed by hospitalists and nonhospitalist community physicians. The study found that, at that

facility, hospitalists averaged less than half the number of handoffs as the community physicians (Bennett 2004).

Conclusion

Hospital leaders will continue to be concerned about the fiscal health of their institutions. Hospitalists have consistently proven in clinical studies that they can bring value to the operation of a healthcare facility. With reduced LOS, decreased overall hospital costs, and equivalent—if not superior—quality, hospitalists can contribute significantly to a hospital's performance.

BENEFIT 6: MAXIMIZING THROUGHPUT AND IMPROVING PATIENT FLOW[7]

Key Message

Hospitalists can positively affect throughput at every stage of the patient care process—emergency department, admission, inpatient unit, surgery, critical care, and discharge.

The issue of throughput, already a concern for many hospital executives, is about to get worse. The senior population—individuals age 65 and older—is projected to experience an 85 percent growth rate over the next two decades. Because this age group uses inpatient services 4.5 times more frequently than do younger populations, the number of admissions and beds needed to accommodate those cases will soar. Currently, the nation's healthcare facilities admit 31 million cases; by 2027, this number will jump to more than 44 million, representing a 41 percent growth from present admissions figures. For hospitals that maintain an 80 percent census rate, an additional 238,000 beds will be needed to meet demands (Solucient 2001).

As practicing clinicians, hospitalists can address throughput on a case-by-case, patient-by-patient basis. However, in a broader sense, hospitalists are inpatient experts who are often asked to lead organization-wide throughput initiatives to identify and implement strategies to facilitate patient flow and efficiency. As dedicated members of multidisciplinary in-house teams, hospitalists are in a prime position to foster change and improve systems.

As illustrated in Table 3.6, hospitalists can positively affect throughput at each stage of the continuum of care, from the emergency department to discharge.

Table 3.6. How Hospitalists Affect Throughput

Stage of Patient Care	Hospitalist Contributions to Improved Throughput
Emergency department	• Potentially improved triaging of patients; accurate classification of the intensity of service • Potentially faster transfer out of the ED
Admission	• 24/7 availability (often on-site) for real-time admission of patients overnight • Availability for care of patients in the observation unit
Inpatient unit	• Effective teamwork and coordination of care, leading to reduced LOS • Ability to rapidly respond to changes in a patient's condition
Surgery	• Comanagement of patients allows the surgeon and the hospitalist to focus on their respective strengths
Intensive care	• Certified hospitalists (advanced cardiac life support and fundamental critical care support certification) meet Leapfrog Group criteria • Facilitation of transfers in and out of the ICU
Discharge	• In-house availability may lead to faster discharge, freeing the bed for a new patient • Familiarity with postcare patient treatment options can result in more rapid discharge

ED: emergency department; LOS: length of stay; ICU: intensive care unit

Conclusion

As hospital administrators attempt to address the issue of expeditiously admitting, treating, and discharging patients in these days of restricted budgets and increased demand, hospitalist programs are poised to be invaluable in the throughput process.

BENEFIT 7: EDUCATING THROUGH FORMAL AND INFORMAL LEARNING PROCESSES[8]

Key Message

Hospitalists are well positioned to educate residents, medical students, patients, physicians, other healthcare professionals, and administrators.

In an inpatient setting, hospitalists can be effective educators. They are capable of analyzing and interpreting a wide range of medical information to treat their patients as well as provide updated information to patients and their families, residents and interns, nursing staff, other healthcare professionals, and hospital administrators. The hospitalist can be viewed as a major resource for educational activities in the inpatient environment by absorbing, synthesizing, and disseminating information.

Dual Educational Tracks

As depicted in Figure 3.2, medical education activity and the ways in which knowledge is imparted fall into two categories: formal and informal. Although some overlap may occur, distinct characteristics are attributable to both classifications.

Formal Education

Formal education refers to the traditional teacher/learner roles in medicine. The learner can be a medical student, a resident, or a fellow. Education is typically transmitted from teacher to learner (as depicted in Figure 3.2 by a solid line), with some reciprocal feedback from the learner to the teacher (dotted line).

Formal education can take place in both academic medical centers and community hospitals. By definition, academic medical centers provide supervised practical training for medical students, student nurses, and/or other healthcare professionals as well as residents and fellows. In many academic medical centers throughout the United States, hospitalists are emerging as core teachers of inpatient medicine.

Figure 3.2. Hospitalists as Inpatient Educators

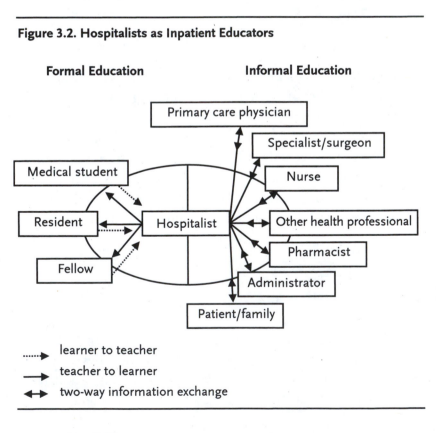

Formal Education · Informal Education

Primary care physician · Specialist/surgeon · Medical student · Nurse · Resident · Hospitalist · Other health professional · Fellow · Pharmacist · Administrator · Patient/family

┄┄▶ learner to teacher
──▶ teacher to learner
◀─▶ two-way information exchange

Community hospitals that have residency programs also incorporate education to some degree into their daily operations. On July 1, 2003, ACGME revised its regulations governing the number of resident duty hours. These changes have forced residency programs to find viable options for imparting the required knowledge and hands-on experience to residents in fewer hours. Many consider hospitalists, by virtue of their "superior clinical and educational skills," as a representation "the solution to the residency work duty problem" (Saint and Flanders 2004).

In 2002, ACGME required six general competencies to be incorporated into residency curriculum and evaluation: patient care, medical knowledge, practice-based learning and improvement, interpersonal and communication skills, professionalism, and systems-based practice. Because their practice already incorporates many aspects of these competencies, hospitalists can be effective at teaching these concepts to residents.

In the formal capacity of teacher, hospitalists can participate in attending and teaching rounds as well as in didactic patient-specific sessions presented in a case-based format, which provides residents with basic knowledge. As teaching supervisors, they can oversee the full range of clinical processes and procedures from the admission stage to the postdischarge stage. Hospitalist teachers can also serve as mentors, providing a role model to residents who may be searching for direction regarding future plans. Through career counseling, hospitalists may steer learners into appropriate areas of study and training. Table 3.7 summarizes research studies that document the positive impact that hospitalists have achieved as formal educators in the academic environment.

Hospitalists may also have formal responsibility for developing curricula for learners in the academic environment. Whether the focus is on teaching medical students, residents, or hospitalist fellows, hospitalists can determine what topics and material need to be covered and then incorporate them into a cogent curriculum.

Table 3.7. Research Results: Hospitalists as Educators

Study Description	Results
University of Chicago Medical Center: resident satisfaction with attending physicians (traditional vs. hospitalist) (Chung et al. 2002)	• In the year-end survey, hospitalists rated higher overall ($p = .05$) and on four measures for "educational environment" • Hospitalists ranked highest for "emphasis on education by attending" ($p < .01$)
Children's Hospital Boston: interns' perception of ward attending physicians (hospitalist vs. nonhospitalist) (Landrigan et al. 2002)	• Mean overall score difference from 4.1 to 4.7 ($p < .01$) for hospitalists vs. nonhospitalists • Significantly higher rankings for hospitalists as teachers and role models • Hospitalist ratings were significantly higher for medical knowledge, accessibility, involvement with the learning process, and feedback
Oregon Health and Science University: medical student evaluations of hospitalist and nonhospitalist faculty (Hunter et al. 2004)	Overall, hospitalist rankings were higher in the following dimensions: • communication of goals • learning climate • teaching style • evaluation and feedback • contributions to student growth/development and overall effectiveness as clinical teacher
Norwalk Hospital, Connecticut: researchers evaluate the effectiveness of hospitalist clinician educators (Kulaga 2004)	• House staff reported changes (compared to previous nonhospitalist model) in behavior on evidence-based medicine and resource utilization • Noted improvements in formal and informal teaching (e.g., bedside rounds, attending rounds, didactic conferences)
Moffitt-Long and Mount Zion Hospitals, San Francisco: two university-affiliated teaching hospitals evaluate hospitalists as inpatient attendings (Hauer et al. 2004)	• Overall satisfaction with hospitalists compared with nonhospitalists was significantly higher (8.3 vs. 8.0 on a 9-point scale; $p < .001$) • Hospitalists received superior ratings as role models in teaching and overall effectiveness, medical knowledge, and interest in teaching • Hospitalists were rated higher in interaction with trainees (i.e., discussing patients and providing feedback)

Informal Education

Informal education can be viewed as an exchange of information among stakeholders in the healthcare industry who are attempting to improve outcomes. Figure 3.2 depicts this as a two-way information exchange (solid arrows in both directions). As hospitalists impart knowledge to PCPs, specialists/surgeons, other healthcare professionals (including nurses and pharmacists), patients, families, and hospital administrators, they reap benefits as well.

This same opportunity for education extends to the hospital floor, where team building serves to enlighten each member of the group providing patient care. In a reciprocal environment, both hospitalists and their medical professional teammates benefit from each other's knowledge.

Hospitalists can initiate informal in-house educational outreach such as informational programs about medical breakthroughs, new medications, existing medical legislation, and other relevant topics. These programs can enlighten nurses, case managers, pharmacists, and other healthcare professionals about issues important to managing patients and/or achieving quality outcomes. The format for these programs may be one-on-one interactions (either in person or by telephone) relating to one specific patient; formal in-service lectures; "Lunch and Learns"; pharmaceutically funded drug or disease management seminars; committee or departmental meetings; and/or random written communications (sent electronically or by interoffice mail) that incorporate history and physical findings, consultations, discharge summaries, or hard-copy articles.

Conclusion

Because they spend so much time in the hospital, hospitalists are positioned to be experts on many aspects of inpatient care—clinical, administrative, patient flow, and healthcare industry issues. Published research shows that academic institutions that employ hospitalist educators are more likely to have more satisfied and better educated students and residents. Likewise, common sense suggests that nurses and other stakeholders who work with hospitalists may be more informed and better educated team members in the patient care process. Hospitalists can be the key ingredient and centerpiece in effective inpatient medical education.

BENEFIT 8: IMPROVING PATIENT SAFETY AND QUALITY OF CARE[9]

Key Message

Hospitalists have the potential to improve quality, resulting in better outcomes, more satisfied patients, and revenue from pay-for-performance contracts.

Since 1999, when the Committee on Quality of Health Care in America of the Institute of Medicine (Kohn, Corrigan, and Donaldson 1999) published its first report, *To Err Is Human: Building a Safer Health System*, patient safety and improved quality of care have become growing priorities for hospital leaders. Consider the following two major trends:

1. *Transparency:* the willingness to publish key quality metrics. A hospital's performance will be available to the public, potentially affecting market share and financial performance.
2. *Pay for performance (P4P):* contracts with payers that include financial incentives based on measurable quality metrics. A hospital's bottom line can be affected by P4P contracts.

Hospitalists as Quality Experts

Many hospital administrators have turned to hospitalists to lead and drive quality and patient safety initiatives in their institutions.

The following attributes of hospitalists make them well qualified for this role:

- Hospitalists, as inpatient experts, are well positioned to integrate hospital systems, thereby maximizing efforts to enhance patient safety. They take care of patients in the hospital every day, so they can examine the processes with which they work. Hospitalists have an ideal perspective from which to reform ineffective systems.
- Effective hospitalists recognize that they are part of a team. By elevating the ideals of teamwork, hospitalists can deliver the essential care that patients need, both while in the hospital and after they are discharged.
- Well-organized hospitalist programs will optimize communication and implement protocols, thus facilitating the practice of delivering safe and consistent care to all patients. With a small, cohesive group of inpatient physicians, the development and implementation of protocols can potentially be more effective than working with a more fragmented group of PCPs.
- A significant portion of a hospitalist's time is spent managing transitions from floor to floor and discharging to home, rehabilitation facility, or nursing home. Each of these transitions presents an opportunity for errors. Effective hospitalists have a thorough understanding of these risks.
- According to a survey conducted by the Society of Hospital Medicine (SHM 2006b), 41 percent of hospital medicine groups have financial incentives relating to measurable quality metrics.

Research Studies

A growing body of research is demonstrating the impact of hospitalists on patient safety and quality of care. Quality of care has been assessed through studies of both process and outcomes of care. Reports of process measures in hospitalist versus traditional inpatient care models for pneumonia, heart failure, end-of-life care, and other conditions have demonstrated that hospitalists improve or maintain quality of care (Lindenauer et al. 2002; Auerbach and Pantilat 2004; Rifkin et al. 2002; Smith, Westfall, and Nicholas 2002). Three studies, one of which was prospective and randomized, have shown improved mortality rate for patients under hospitalist care versus traditional care (Meltzer et al. 2002; Auerbach et al. 2002; Tenner et al. 2003). At least one study indicated a decrease in 30-day readmission rates (Kulaga 2004). In summarizing the research to date, quality of care is at least as good, and is possibly improved, under hospitalists. However, more studies are needed to conclusively say that hospitalists provide more superior quality compared to the traditional care model.

Conclusion

Patient safety and quality of care in the hospital require a team of dedicated people to effect change. With the numerous handoffs that take place during hospitalization, the potential for medical errors increases exponentially. A well-organized hospitalist program can play a significant role in orchestrating the team effectively.

NOTES

1. This material has been adapted from Society of Hospital Medicine Benchmarks Committee and P. Hanlon. 2005. "How Hospitalists Add Value: Treating Unassigned Patients." *The Hospitalist* 9 (suppl. 1): 8–10.

2. This material has been adapted from Society of Hospital Medicine Benchmarks Committee, M. Pak, K. Kerr, and P. Hanlon. 2005. "How Hospitalists Add Value: Leading Medical Staffs." *The Hospitalist* 9 (suppl. 1): 11–13.

3. The term "physician home team" is often used by Laurence Wellikson, M.D., chief executive officer at Society of Hospital Medicine.

4. This material has been adapted from Society of Hospital Medicine Benchmarks Committee, B. T. Kealey, L. Vidrine, and P. Hanlon. 2005. "How Hospitalists Add Value: Improving Physicians' Practices." *The Hospitalist* 9 (suppl. 1): 14–17.

5. This material has been adapted from Society of Hospital Medicine Benchmarks Committee, S. Goldsholl, and P. Hanlon. 2005. "How Hospitalists Add Value: Providing Extraordinary Availability." *The Hospitalist* 9 (suppl. 1): 18–21.

6. This material has been adapted from Society of Hospital Medicine Benchmarks Committee, S. Syed, and P. Hanlon. 2005. "How Hospitalists Add Value: Improving Resource Utilization." *The Hospitalist* 9 (suppl. 1): 22–25.

7. This material has been adapted from Society of Hospital Medicine Benchmarks Committee, P. Cawley, and P. Hanlon. 2005. "How Hospitalists Add Value: Maximizing Throughput and Improving Patient Flow." *The Hospitalist* 9 (suppl. 1): 26–28.

8. This material has been adapted from Society of Hospital Medicine Benchmarks Committee, M. Pak, T. Jones, and P. Hanlon. 2005. "How Hospitalists Add Value: Educating Through Formal and Informal Learning Processes." *The Hospitalist* 9 (suppl. 1): 29–32.

9. This material has been adapted from Society of Hospital Medicine Benchmarks Committee, M. Pak, and P. Hanlon. 2005. "How Hospitalists Add Value: Improving Patient Safety and Quality of Care." *The Hospitalist* 9 (suppl. 1): 33–35.

REFERENCES

Appleby, J. 1999. "Hospitals Plagued by On-Call Shortage," *USA Today*, June 16.

Auerbach, A. D., E. A. Nelson, P. K. Lindenauer, S. Z. Pantilat, P. P. Katz, and R. M. Wachter. 2000. "Physician Attitudes Toward and Prevalence of the Hospitalist Model of Care: Results of a National Survey." *American Journal of Medicine* 109 (8): 648–53.

Auerbach, A. D., R. M. Wachter, P. Katz, J. Showstack, R. B. Baron, and L. Goldman. 2002. "Implementation of a Voluntary Hospitalist Service at a Community Teaching Hospital: Improved Clinical Efficiency and Patient Outcomes." *Annals of Internal Medicine* 137 (11): 859–65.

Auerbach, A. D., M. D. Aronson, R. B. Davis, and R. S. Phillips. 2003. "How Physicians Perceive Hospitalist Services After Implementation: Anticipation vs. Reality." *Archives of Internal Medicine* 163 (19): 2330–36.

Auerbach, A. D., and S. Z. Pantilat. 2004. "End of Life Care in a Voluntary Hospitalist Model: Effects on Communication, Processes of Care, and Patient Symptoms." *American Journal of Medicine* 116 (10): 669–75.

Bennett, Adrienne, M.D., chief of hospitalist service, Newton-Wellesley Hospital, Newton, MA. 2004. Telephone interview, December 15.

Chung, P., J. Morrison, L. Jin, W. Levinson, H. Humphrey, and D. Meltzer. 2002. "Resident Satisfaction on an Academic Hospitalist Service: Time to Teach." *American Journal of Medicine* 112 (7): 597–601.

Everett, G. D., M. P. Anton, B. K. Jackson, C. Swigert, and N. Uddin. 2004. "Comparison of Hospital Costs and Length of Stay Associated with General Internists and Hospitalist Physicians at a Community Hospital." *American Journal of Managed Care* 10 (9): 626–30.

Fernandez, A., K. Grumbach, L. Grotein, K. Vranizan, H. Osmond, and A. B. Bindman. 2000. "Friend or Foe? How Primary Care Physicians Perceive Hospitalists." *Archives of Internal Medicine* 160 (19): 2902–8.

Foubister, V. 1999. "Is There a Dearth of Specialists in the ED?" *American Medical News* (July 12): 42.

Gregory, D., W. Baigelman, and I. B. Wilson. 2003. "Hospital Economics of the Hospitalist." *Health Services Research* 38 (3): 905–18; discussion 919–22.

Halpert, A. P., S. D. Pearson, H. E. LeWine, S. C. McKean. 2000. "The Impact of an Inpatient Physician Program on Quality, Utilization, and Satisfaction." *American Journal of Managed Care* 6 (5): 549–55.

Hauer, K. E., R. M. Wachter, C. E. McCulloch, G. A. Woo, and A. D. Auerbach. 2004. "Effects of Hospitalist Attending Physicians on Trainee Satisfaction with Teaching and with Internal Medicine Rotations." *Archives of Internal Medicine* 164: 1866–71.

Huddleston, J. M., K. H. Long, J. M. Naessens, D. Vanness, D. Larson, R. Trousdale, M. Plevak, M. Cabanela, D. Ilstrup, and R. M. Wachter. 2004. "Medical and Surgical Comanagement After Elective Hip and Knee Arthroplasty: A Randomized, Controlled Trial." *Annals of Internal Medicine* 141 (1): 28–38.

Hunter, A. J., S. S. Desai, R. A. Harrison, and B. K. Chen. 2004. "Medical Student Evaluation of the Quality of Hospitalist and Non-Hospitalist Teaching Faculty on Inpatient Medicine Rotations." *Academic Medicine* 79 (1): 78–82.

Jackson, C. 2001. "Doctors Find Hospitalists Save Time, Money: Primary Care Physicians Are Seeing that Turning Over Their Hospital Business Allows Them to Make More Income." [Online article; retrieved 02/17/07.] www.ama-assn.org/amed-news.

Kaboli, P. J., M. J. Barnett, and G. E. Rosenthal. 2004. "Associations with Reduced Length of Stay and Costs on an Academic Hospitalist Service." *American Journal of Managed Care* 10 (8): 561–68.

Kohn, L. T., J. M. Corrigan, and M. S. Donaldson (eds.). 1999. *To Err Is Human: Building a Safer Health System.* Washington, DC: National Academies Press.

Kulaga, M. E. 2004. "The Positive Impact of Initiation of Hospitalist Clinician Educators." *Journal of General Internal Medicine* 19 (4): 293–301.

Landrigan, C. P., S. Muret-Wagstaff, V. W. Chiang, D. J. Nigrin, D. A. Goldmann, and J. A. Finkelstein. 2002. "Effect of a Pediatric Hospitalist System on Housestaff Education and Experience." *Archives of Pediatrics and Adolescent Medicine* 156 (9): 877–83.

Landro, L. 2004. "Medicine's Fastest-Growing Specialty: Hospital-Bound Doctors Take the Place of Your Physician; Effort to Reduce Costs, Errors." [Online article; retrieved 01/28/07] http://online.wsj.com/public/us.

Lindenauer, P. K., R. Chehabbeddine, P. Pekow, J. Fitzgerald, and E. M. Benjamin. 2002. "Quality of Care for Patients Hospitalized with Heart Failure: Assessing the Impact of Hospitalists." *Archives of Internal Medicine* 162 (11): 1251–56.

Massey, B. 2004. "Trendy Hospital Medicine Comes to Charlotte." *Charlotte Sun*, February 13.

McGowan, R. A. 2006. "Strategies for Strengthening Physician-Hospital Alignment: A National Study." Chicago: Society for Healthcare Strategy and Market Development of the American Hospital Association and Mitretek Systems, Inc.

————. 2004. "Strengthening Hospital-Physician Relationships." *Healthcare Financial Management* 58 (12): 38–42.

Meltzer, D., W. Manning, J. Morrison, M. Shah, L. Jiu, T. Guth, and W. Levinson. 2002. "Effects of Physician Experience on Costs and Outcomes on an Academic General Medical Service: Results of a Trial of Hospitalists." *Annals of Internal Medicine* 137 (11): 866–74.

Palmer, H. C., Jr., N. S. Armistead, P. M. Elnicki, A. K. Halperin, P. R. Opershok, S. Manivannan, G. R. Hobbs, and K. Evans. 2001. "The Effect of a Hospitalist Service with Nurse Discharge Planner on Patient Care in an Academic Teaching Hospital." *American Journal of Medicine* 111 (8): 627–32.

Rifkin, W. D., D. Conner, A. Silver, and A. Eichorn. 2002. "Comparison of Processes and Outcomes of Pneumonia Care Between Hospitalists and Community-based Primary Care Physicians." *Mayo Clinic Proceedings* 77 (10): 1053–58.

Saint, S., and S. A. Flanders. 2004. "Hospitalists in Teaching Hospitals: Opportunities But Not Without Danger." *Journal of General Internal Medicine* 19 (4): 392–93.

Smith, P. C., J. M. Westfall, and R. A. Nicholas. 2002. "Primary Care Family Physicians and 2 Hospitalist Models: Comparison of Outcomes, Processes, and Costs." *Journal of Family Practice* 51 (12): 1021–27.

Society of Hospital Medicine (SHM). 2006a. *2005–2006 SHM Survey: State of the Hospital Medicine Movement.* Philadelphia, PA: Society of Hospital Medicine.

————. 2006b. SHM Special Issues Survey. Philadelphia, PA: Society of Hospital Medicine.

Solucient. 2001. "National and Local Impact of Long-Term Demographic Change on Inpatient Acute Care." Evanston, IL: Solucient.

Taylor, M. 1999. "Blaming the Docs: Patient Dumping Probes See Physicians as Culprits in Turning Away Indigent from ERs." *Modern Healthcare* 29 (32): 36–38.

Tenner, P. A., H. Dibrell, R. P. Taylor, and P. Richard. 2003. "Improved Survival with Hospitalists in a Pediatric Intensive Care Unit." *Critical Care Medicine* 31 (3): 847–52.

Wachter, R. M., and L. Goldman. 2002. "The Hospitalist Movement Five Years Later." *Journal of the American Medical Association* 287 (4): 487–94.

Winston, K., and the Advisory Board Company Clinical Initiatives Center. 2000. "Cause for Concern: Ensuring Adequate and Timely On-Call Physician Coverage in the Emergency Department." *ED Watch* Issue #4, May 2.

CHAPTER 4

What Is the Return on Investment for Hospitalists?

Key Message

Hospital administrators should conduct a formal financial analysis of their hospitalist programs, examining revenues, expenses, and return on investment (ROI). It is reasonable to expect as much as a 2-to-1 or 3-to-1 ROI.

With rare exceptions, hospitalist programs are not financially viable solely on the basis of professional-fee revenue. They nearly always require additional financial support, which usually comes from the hospital in which they work or some other sponsoring organization, such as a large medical group or healthcare network. There are several reasons that professional-fee collections alone are not enough to support most practices:

- Most practices care for a large number of unassigned patients (i.e., those without a primary care physician) admitted from the emergency department, which can mean a poor payer mix.
- In many practices, there is enough night work to require additional staffing, but the opportunity to generate professional-fee revenue from that night work is often limited.

- Hospitalist practices typically experience variations in patient volume from one day to the next that are more significant than in most other physician practices. Little opportunity exists to schedule patient visits as efficiently as can be done in an office practice. Thus, an individual hospitalist might generate fees efficiently for only part of each working day.
- Traditionally, professional-fee revenues for inpatient, nonprocedural care (the vast majority of a hospitalist's billings) have been low. Until 2007, reform efforts to bolster nonprocedural reimbursement for physicians have focused almost entirely on office care.
- Demand for hospitalists has consistently outstripped the availability of doctors, which contributes to hospitalist incomes being higher than fee collections.

Because hospitalists require financial support, hospital administrators must be sure that their institution is receiving sufficient value for their investment. Consider the following data from the Society of Hospital Medicine's (SHM 2006) biannual survey on the state of the hospitalist movement:

- 97 percent of hospital medicine groups receive financial support from one or more outside sources (in addition to collections from professional fees). The sources are as follows:
  o Hospital—94 percent
  o Physician organization/group practice—9 percent
  o Medical school/academic institution—13 percent
  o Other—4 percent
- The median deficit for hospital medicine groups is $550,000, which represents 25 to 30 percent of the group's total income.
- Financial support averages approximately $60,000 per full-time equivalent hospitalist.

A formal financial analysis of a hospitalist program should examine four dimensions:

1. Projected revenues
2. Projected expenses
3. Projected deficit (i.e., amount of financial support required)
4. Financial benefits of the program

By comparing the financial benefits of the program to the amount of financial support required, a return on investment (ROI) can be computed.

PROJECTED REVENUES

Although other revenue sources may be available (e.g., grants), the primary revenue source for hospitalists is professional-fee collections. Often, hospital medicine groups fail to maximize their professional-fee collections because of one or more of the following reasons:

- No production incentives are in place for hospitalists.
- Hospitalists do not capture and report all charges.
- Hospitalists do not adequately document codes and/or select the appropriate code.
- The billing service does not provide adequate billing reports.
- The billing service does not recognize that hospitalists deliver a different level of service (when compared to community physicians).
- The billing service does an inadequate job of collections.

In developing a financial analysis of a hospital medicine group, benchmarks from SHM's 2006 survey provide a useful perspective (see Table 4.1). The following factors are key to understanding the survey findings:

- *Region.* Hospitalists in the South region had the highest collections (median $194,000 per hospitalist per year), 18 percent higher than those in the East region, which had the lowest

Table 4.1. Benchmarks on Hospitalist Charges and Collections

Type of Hospitalist	Charges (Median)	Collections (Median)	Collection Rate (Median)
All physician hospitalists	$324,000	$183,000	56%
East	$311,000	$164,000	53%
South	$354,000	$194,000	55%
Midwest	$323,000	$192,000	59%
West	$298,000	$175,000	59%
Less than one year as a hospitalist	$275,000	$140,000	51%
Four or more years as a hospitalist	$372,000	$182,000	49%
Salary only	$276,000	$150,000	54%
Productivity/performance compensation only	$392,000	$231,000	59%
Mix: salary plus productivity/performance compensation (or bonus)	$333,000	$189,000	57%
General internist	$331,000	$189,000	57%
General pediatrician	$251,000	$119,000	47%
Hospital employee	$332,000	$167,000	50%
Local, private hospitalist-only group	$345,000	$200,000	58%
Multistate hospitalist-only group or management company	$343,000	$315,000	92%
Multispecialty/primary care group	$347,000	$200,000	58%
Academic: teaching service	$298,000	$122,000	41%
Academic: combination teaching/nonteaching	$275,000	$120,000	44%

Source: SHM (2006).

collections (median $164,000). Hospitalists in the East had the lowest collection rate (53 percent), perhaps because they had more academic hospitalists.

- *Years as a hospitalist.* Hospitalists with four or more years of experience collected a median of $182,000 per year, 30 percent more than hospitalists with less than one year of experience (median $140,000).
- *Compensation model.* Hospitalists compensated based on a pure productivity/performance basis collected the most (median $231,000). This is 54 percent higher than the collections by salaried hospitalists (median $150,000). Hospitalists compensated on a mix of salary and bonus fell in the middle (median $189,000). The hospitalists compensated on pure performance/productivity also had the highest collection rate (59 percent).
- *Specialty.* General internists had median collections of $189,000 per year, 59 percent more than pediatric hospitalists (median $119,000).
- *Employment model.* Private practice hospitalists collected the most. Multistate hospitalist-only groups/management companies had a median of $315,000 and a collection rate of 92 percent, multispecialty/primary care groups had a median of $200,000 and a collection rate of 58 percent, and local hospitalist-only groups had a median of $200,000 and a collection rate of 58 percent. At the other end of the spectrum, academic hospitalists had the lowest collections. Academic: teaching service had a median of $122,000 and a collection rate of 41 percent, and academic: combination teaching and nonteaching had a median of $120,000 and a collection rate of 44 percent.

Another potential revenue source for hospitalist programs is pay-for-performance (P4P) contracts. Increasingly, health plans are implementing contracts with hospitals that include financial incentives based on quality metrics. Medicare is actively implementing a version of P4P for hospitals. Hospital administrators may want to consider partnering with their hospitalists for P4P. Hospitalists often are responsible for a significant proportion of the hospital's medical admissions. This relatively small, cohesive group of physicians can have a significant impact on quality performance and the hospital's P4P revenue opportunities. Also, in July 2007, Medicare implemented a physician pay-for-reporting program, called the Physician Quality Reporting Initiative, that will most likely evolve into a P4P program over time.

PROJECTED EXPENSES

On average, according to the SHM 2006 survey, staff compensation and benefits account for 80 percent of the expenses of a hospital medicine group. Benchmarks on compensation and benefits from the survey (see Table 4.2) provide a useful perspective for conducting a financial analysis of a hospital medicine group.

The prominent factors in compensation and benefits benchmarks are as follows:

- *Region.* Physician hospitalists in the South were the highest paid—12 percent higher than those in the West, the lowest-paid region (median $205,900 versus $184,000, respectively).
- *Years as a hospitalist.* Physician hospitalists with four or more years of experience earned 22 percent more than those who have less than one year of experience (median $208,000 versus $170,000, respectively).
- *Specialty.* Total compensation for general internists averaged 20 percent more than hospitalists who are general pediatricians (median $197,000 versus $164,000, respectively).
- *Employment model.* At a median of $209,250, physician hospitalists who work for multispecialty/primary care medical groups were the highest paid, at 23 percent more than academic hospitalists who work on a teaching service (median $170,000).

Table 4.2. Hospitalist Compensation and Benefits Benchmarks

Type of Hospitalist	Compensation (Median)	Benefits (Median)	Total
All physician hospitalists	$169,000	$27,000	$196,000
East	$162,000	$28,000	$190,000
South	$180,000	$25,900	$205,900
Midwest	$165,000	$31,000	$196,000
West	$164,000	$20,000	$184,000
Less than one year as a hospitalist	$150,000	$20,000	$170,000
Four or more years as a hospitalist	$178,000	$30,000	$208,000
General internist	$171,000	$26,600	$197,600
General pediatrician	$139,000	$25,000	$164,000
Hospital employee	$172,000	$27,388	$199,388
Local, private hospitalist-only group	$166,000	$33,000	$199,000
Multistate hospitalist-only group or management company	$168,000	$14,138	$182,138
Multispecialty/primary care group	$178,000	$31,250	$209,250
Academic: teaching service	$142,000	$28,000	$170,000
Academic: combination teaching/nonteaching	$153,000	$30,030	$183,030

Source: SHM (2006).

FINANCIAL BENEFITS

As discussed in Chapter 3, research has demonstrated that hospitalists consistently achieve measurable reductions in length of stay and cost per stay. In estimating the financial benefits of this utilization performance, the hospital chief financial officer and finance staff need to provide the following:

- Accurate identification of hospitalist cases
- Net patient revenue (actual collections per case)
- Actual costs of care, including both direct and indirect costs
  - o Note: If the hospital does not have the cost accounting tools to provide these actual costs, a ratio of costs to charges can be used
- Case-mix adjustment
- A comparison group—typically the department of medicine or pediatrics (excluding hospitalists)

Table 4.3 illustrates an actual example of a financial analysis for a hospital medicine group at a community hospital in the midwestern United States.

Table 4.3. Calculation of Return on Investment: Example 1

	Hospitalist (1,514 Cases)	Internal Medicine (2,630 Cases)
1. Net patient revenue	$10,017,000	$18,353,000
2. Direct cost	$5,724,000	$11,681,000
A. Direct cost per case	$3,781	$4,441
B. CMA direct cost per case	$2,996	$3,495
3. Direct cost CMA savings per case (vs. IM)	$499	N/A
4. Direct cost CMA savings total (vs. IM)	$755,000	N/A
5. Indirect cost	$3,218,000	$6,889,000
6. Total cost (item 2 + item 5)	$8,942,000	$18,570,000
7. Net income (item 1 − item 6)	$1,075,000	($217,000)
Net income per case	$710	($83)

CMA: case-mix adjusted; IM: internal medicine; N/A; not applicable

Source: Goldsholl (2007).

In example 1, provided in Table 4.3, the following should be noted:

- Compared to the internal medicine physicians, the hospitalist program saved the hospital $499 in direct costs per case (on a case-mix adjusted basis), or $755,000 in total.
- The hospitalist program was "profitable," contributing more than $1 million to the hospital's bottom line (compared to the internal medicine physicians, whose cases generated more than $200,000 in losses for the hospital).

This hospital invested $300,000 in the hospital medicine group, covering the program's deficit. The ROI for the hospitalists was more than 3 to 1 ($1 million vs. $300,000).

Another potential source of financial benefit to the hospital is derived from the fact that reducing length of stay results in increased throughput and the potential for the hospital to service additional cases. Some of those additional cases may be more profitable (e.g., surgical cases), resulting in additional contributions to the hospital's bottom line.

At the SHM Annual Meeting in 2002, Robert M. Wachter, M.D., associate chair in the department of medicine at the University of California, San Francisco, presented an ROI analysis of a hospitalist program at a large university teaching hospital (see Table 4.4).

Table 4.4. Calculation of Return on Investment: Example 2

Analysis of the Hospitalist Program at a Large University

1,950 patients × $1,571 (savings/patient)	$3,063,450
Add 1,092 bed days saved × $500 (estimated cost per bed-day)	$ 546,000
Total annual benefit to medical center	$3,609,450
2000–2001 medical center funding	$ 625,000
Return on investment	>$3.6 million for $625,000 investment

Source: Wachter (2002).

The analysis concludes that an ROI of 5.8 to 1 ($3.6 million in benefits on an investment of $625,000) was achieved. The financial benefit includes an estimate of $546,000 in contribution to the bottom line from 1,092 bed days saved, each at the rate of $500.

In addition to cost-per-stay savings and throughput contributions to the bottom line, the following list documents other potential benefits of a hospitalist program. Not all of the benefits can be easily quantified from a financial perspective.

- Reduced number of decertification denials
- Improved responsiveness to emergency patients
- Increased satisfaction of the nursing staff
- Effective utilization of specialists
- Reduced burden of emergency call on primary care physicians
- Better coordination with case management and discharge planning
- Increased referrals from surrounding markets
- Ability to attract and retain primary care physicians

CONCLUSION

Hospitalist programs nearly always require financial support in addition to collected professional-fee revenue, but they have the potential to generate substantial benefits. Hospital administrators should work with the hospitalist medical director to instill financial discipline so that performing an ROI analysis becomes a routine exercise.

REFERENCES

Goldsholl, S. 2007. "The Hospitalist Dashboard: A Case Study in the Power of Data." Presentation at the Society of Hospital Medicine Annual Meeting, Dallas, TX, May 23.

Society of Hospital Medicine (SHM). 2006. *2005–2006 SHM Survey: State of the Hospital Medicine Movement.* Philadelphia, PA: Society of Hospital Medicine.

Wachter, R. M. 2002. "Making the Case: Creating Value and Demonstrating It to Others." Presentation at the Society of Hospital Medicine Annual Meeting, Philadelphia, PA, April 9.

CHAPTER 5

Hospitalist Program Essentials: Achieving Success and Avoiding Failure

Key Message

The top essentials for building a successful hospitalist program include picking the right leader, implementing incentive compensation, designing an effective schedule, focusing on recruiting, developing a proficiency in coding, and measuring performance against goals.

A number of factors increase the likelihood that a hospitalist program will fail. These factors include poor leadership, underestimating patient-volume growth, failing to create a practice-owner mentality, excessive overhead, setting inappropriate expectations, excessive workload, and insufficient financial support.

ACHIEVING SUCCESS

As the hospitalist movement has evolved, a body of knowledge is developing regarding the key elements necessary to start up a new hospitalist practice or to improve an existing one. These keys to success have been summarized as the top ten hospitalist program essentials for hospital executives. The list provides a set of conditions for a successful program. Although addressing these ten essentials should improve performance, ultimately a complex interplay of factors will determine success or failure. The items have not been ranked because their relative importance can change significantly from one practice to the next. But experience has shown that every practice should be thinking about all ten essentials.

1. Pick the Right Leader

Selecting the right leader is fundamental to a successful practice. These individuals are hard to find. They must be excellent clinically and have superb communication skills. Although they need to be assertive, they must also be good listeners. Political skills are essential to navigate medical staff, departmental, and administrative issues. An understanding of and appreciation for practice economics will help to ensure that revenue is optimized and benefits to the hospital are tracked. The leader should have some reduction in clinical time compared with the other full-time doctors in the practice (5 percent reduction in clinical time for every full-time equivalent doctor in the group is a reasonable rule of thumb). Chapter 14 addresses the role of the hospitalist medical director.

2. Implement Incentive Compensation

While a fixed salary can be attractive to many hospitalists and may facilitate recruiting, it often becomes a significant hindrance to optimal practice operation. A compensation system that rewards performance is preferable. The goal of the compensation should be to connect physician incomes with the economic health and/or clinical quality of the practice. In this way, doctors will think of themselves as owners of their practice (even if they are employees of a hospital or a multispecialty clinic) and not just employees who feel like it is someone else's problem to address the financial status of the program.

Production-based incentives (e.g., based on work relative value units [wRVUs]) can be an effective way to achieve this goal. Each hospitalist can make personal choices about how much she wants to work and accept the economic consequences of that decision. While hospitalists may view production-based compensation as a way to make them work too hard, it can instead be liberating for each doctor, linking work output to financial reward and reducing the need for each doctor to have nearly identical workloads. Society of Hospital Medicine (SHM 2006) survey data indicate that hospitalists who are compensated based on some type of production incentive earn 13 percent more and generate 18 percent more RVUs annually than those who do not have a production component to their compensation. Note that quality-based incentives (e.g., based on Joint Commission core measures) can also lead to positive performance and are a growing trend among hospitalists. See Chapter 13 for a more extensive discussion of compensation.

3. Design a Thoughtful, Flexible Physician Schedule

A hospitalist's schedule should take into account the following variables:

- *Patient–hospitalist continuity over the course of the hospital stay.* Ideally, a patient should see the same hospitalist throughout his hospital stay. This is likely to improve patient satisfaction, reduce errors, and increase hospitalist efficiency. Hospitalists should typically work as many consecutive days as is reasonable for their lifestyle.
- *Sustainable physician lifestyle.* Is the group's schedule one that a doctor could work for many years? Or do problems arise, such as regular night work, leading to sleep deprivation or working too few days annually so that each worked day requires a very high patient load?
- *Reasonable provision for night work.* Once a hospitalist group is admitting six to eight patients per day, the program should

consider a separate night shift staffed by a doctor who has no daytime responsibility the day before or after. Ideally, the practice should have one or more dedicated "nocturnists" who work only at night, while the remaining doctors in the group work only during the daytime.

- *Adaptability and scalability.* Every group should think about how their schedule might change if or when patient volume grows and one or more doctors are added. Growth will often require changing the schedule significantly, rather than just adding new doctors into the existing scheduling rotation. For example, a group following a 7-on/7-off schedule (half the doctors work each week, and the other half are off) that needs to add one more doctor will require substantial changes to the schedule.

See Chapter 11 for a broader discussion on scheduling.

4. Plan for Day-to-Day Variations in Patient Volume

It is important to anticipate daily fluctuations in patient volume and have some plan in place for handling these fluctuations. No simple strategy exists to deal with this issue, but ways can be found to mitigate the problem. The following are some ideas to consider:

- *Implement a patient volume cap for individual hospitalists.* A cap on volume for an individual doctor in the practice can be valuable. This would mean that when one doctor reaches the cap, other hospitalists help out. But it is best to avoid a patient volume cap for the whole practice that requires nonhospitalists to begin helping out when the hospitalists are capped. An exception to this rule is academic teaching hospitals, which have a mandated volume cap for the whole practice that is based on residency requirements.

- *Deploy human resources to reflect the bimodal distribution in work over the course of the day.* A typical hospitalist practice is very busy with rounds on existing patients from early in the morning until sometime in the early afternoon. Then it is busy with admissions from early afternoon until about 10 p.m. to midnight. Larger practices (e.g., 15 or more admissions daily) may want to consider dividing the day's staffing into several doctors who round and admit during the working day and have a different doctor(s) come on duty to handle late-evening and night admissions.
- *Avoid daytime shifts with rigid start and stop times.* It is unlikely that the day's patient volume will be consistent from day to day, week to week. Hospitalists should acknowledge that the number of hours they work on a particular day is a function of the patient volume rather than predetermined shifts. While this type of scheduling can mean working longer than average on some days, it also means that when patient volume is low, some hospitalists can leave early rather than wait until the end of a predetermined shift.
- *Avoid doctors on "jeopardy" who are called in from home if the practice gets busy.* This is usually not an effective system. Busy doctors are often reluctant to call in the jeopardy doctor, because next week the roles may be reversed and they do not want to be called in while on jeopardy. It is usually better for the regularly scheduled doctors to work longer days (within reason) than to identify someone to be available at all times from home.

5. Never Stop Recruiting

A significant problem encountered by many if not most new hospitalist programs is patient-volume growth that occurs more quickly than anticipated. Recruiting lead times for hospitalists are long, and physician turnover is common. A frequent cause of hospitalist practice crisis or failure is an overwhelmed hospitalist team. Unexpectedly high volumes lead to stress and turnover, only exacerbating the problem for the remaining physicians. The key to minimizing this stress is to maintain an active recruitment effort supported by a competitive compensation program. This can be outsourced to a search firm, maintained in-house, or handled through some combination of both. Developing a close relationship with nearby residency programs can be valuable. Appendix B contains recommendations for developing a recruiting strategy.

6. Anticipate Ongoing Evolution in the Scope of Practice

Hospitalists should expect to assume a broader set of responsibilities than primary care physicians practicing in the inpatient environment. During residency, most internists did not think of themselves as the attending physician of record for patients with hip fracture, for example. But many hospitals see value in having a hospitalist comanage these patients, which in some cases may include serving as the attending physician of record. All hospitalists should be prepared for an evolving set of responsibilities that may increasingly expand beyond the traditional scope of their training background. They should work diligently to acquire the needed skills and expertise.

7. Track and Report Performance Measures Against Goals

Ideally, the practice's business plan should establish an initial set of performance goals and metrics. But in a rush to get up and running, many hospitalist practices fail to do this. By tracking performance against these measures, variations can be picked up earlier in the process and corrective actions introduced. Many programs wait 6 to 12 months to examine program performance when corrective actions may face more entrenched behaviors. Instead, hospitalists should be provided with quarterly or monthly reports of their performance on many parameters such as clinical quality, resource utilization, practice economics, physician productivity, and satisfaction (of patients, referring physicians, nurses, and hospitalists). Performance measurement is discussed in Chapter 15.

8. Ensure that Hospitalists Are Proficient in Documentation and Coding

Poor coding, especially undercoding, is a common problem among hospitalist programs. This is especially true for programs that have not implemented production-based incentives. Educating the doctors in coding and undertaking regular audits of their performance are worth the effort and expense. These actions can lead to significant additional revenue to the hospitalist practice, potentially reducing the amount of financial support required from the hospital. See Chapter 17 for a more detailed discussion of billing and coding.

9. Select an Experienced Billing and Collections Agency

Unless patient encounters are coded properly, billed accurately and promptly, and collected fully, the hospitalist practice will experience significant deficits and/or require excessive levels of subsidization. Hospital billing departments typically are not familiar with the role of hospitalists. Seek out a vendor that has experience in the hospitalist field and check its references. Make sure it has integrated a compliance program into the coding and billing process and has the ability to provide complete activity and trend reports. Typical expenses for such a service range from 8 percent to 12 percent of collections.

Be sure to audit the firm's performance as well. The audit can be as simple as randomly selecting 10 to 15 patients and going through the billing records to ensure that all charges were posted correctly, attributed to the correct doctor, and pursued until paid or written off according to mutually agreed-upon criteria.

10. Develop a Communications Plan

Communication with referral sources, typically primary care physicians, on admission and discharge should be well organized and consistently executed. Admission and discharge notes should be dictated at the time the patient is seen and then transcribed and transmitted to the referring doctor on a "stat" basis. Telephone contact between the hospitalist and the primary care physician can be valuable in some situations, such as for a new hospitalist practice or any time unique issues arise regarding clinical decisions or significant unexpected changes in a patient's condition. In addition, the communications plan should establish internal operating guidelines for response times by the practice to pages, phone inquiries, and consultation requests. The development of a communications plan is discussed in Chapter 9.

Hospitalists should provide a printed brochure that introduces patients to the individual doctors and describes the concept of hospitalist practice. (See Appendix C for a sample brochure.) Additionally, many hospitalists have found that telephone contact between the hospitalist and the patient after discharge can be valuable in ensuring clinical quality and patient satisfaction. Also, it can be valuable to provide patients with copies of the discharge summaries as they leave the hospital or by mail a few days later.

AVOIDING FAILURE

So far this chapter has highlighted some of the most important issues for hospital executives to get right when developing and maintaining a hospitalist program. This section shares seven common pitfalls that plague hospitalist practices, which can lead to the collapse of some practices. The collapse of a hospital medicine group may not always be the end of hospitalists at a hospital. Failure of a hospitalist practice most often results in a vigorous effort to start over, accompanied by increased resolve and resources to "get it right this time."

While these issues may not cause the failure of a whole practice, they are likely to result in hospitalist dissatisfaction and/or major concerns by the hospital executive team.

1. Instituting Poor Leadership

Because of time pressure, many hospitalist practices start up with doctors who do not have any prior hospitalist experience. This approach may result in a physician leader who is poorly suited for the role. For a practice that is uncertain whether an appropriate medical director can be found among the initial doctors hired, it may be a good idea to wait a year or two to select the leader. An interim leadership model can be implemented taking advantage of physician leaders in the hospital (e.g., the vice president of medical affairs, respected primary care physicians, or emergency physicians). Also, establishing a hospitalist oversight committee composed of leaders of the medical staff can provide guidance to the new program.

2. Underestimating How Rapidly Patient Volume Will Grow

This is among the most common mistakes made by new hospitalist practices. The first few doctors in the practice can become worn out and may quit. This has led to the collapse of some practices. Because of recruiting cycles that can last many months, it is important to continue recruiting, even before a clear need for additional staff has been demonstrated. For most practices, this means they should never stop recruiting.

3. Employing Hospitalists Who Do Not Have a Practice-Owner Mentality

Many doctors seek work as hospitalists to avoid the complexity, commitment, and pressures of outpatient practice. But practicing inpatient medicine is also demanding, and hospitalists do not typically work traditional hours (Monday to Friday, daytime) all the time. For these reasons, hospitalist practices tend to attract doctors who simply want to see patients and leave management of the practice and its financial health to others. This tendency may be exacerbated in practices that compensate hospitalists in a way that is not connected to the overall financial health of the practice (e.g., a straight salary).

This mentality can create a culture among hospitalists in which they think their job is only to see the next patient. They may be reluctant to participate in efforts to ensure the financial health of the practice. For example, they may not be attentive to optimal documentation and coding, and the practice may lose significant billing revenue; they may not want to accept new referrals or see growth in the practice; or they may be too quick to add doctors to the group, thereby working less.

Even if the doctors are employees (of a hospital or other large entity), every effort should be made to encourage them to think of themselves as owners of their practice. The best way to create this environment is to have a tight connection between the economic health of the practice and the hospitalists' income (e.g., via production-based incentive compensation). This should lead to greater autonomy in decision making and hospitalist satisfaction.

4. Carrying Excessive or Inappropriate Hospitalist Overhead

Overhead issues can take two forms:

1. *Excessive overhead* results from a practice of securing too much office space and/or staff support. Because the majority of a

hospitalist's work is done on hospital wards, it is usually sufficient for a hospitalist group to share a single office with seating and workstations (e.g., computers) for one-third to one-half of the total number of doctors in the group (e.g., a 12-hospitalist group might share an office with four to six workstations). A small group (e.g., six or fewer doctors) might do fine with a single clerical assistant who supports the hospitalist and some other department at the same time.

2. *Inappropriate overhead* may occur in multispecialty groups that add hospitalists and charge them the same overhead that the office physicians pay. This high overhead rate (often more than 50 percent) may leave insufficient funds to pay the hospitalists a competitive salary. Thus, it is important for the group to assess hospitalists' overhead based on the resources they actually consume. This would usually include the cost of billing and collections, malpractice insurance, and modest clerical support. The hospitalist collections should not ordinarily go to support office-based expenses of support staff and building/equipment expenses.

5. Allowing Inappropriate Expectations of Hospitalists

To gain support from the medical staff in the early stages of a program, hospitalists can overcommit, assuming responsibility for "scut work"—services that are unattractive to perform. This is not a sustainable model. Eventually, it will be hard to tell other physicians that they must take back responsibility for work the hospitalists have been doing. This is likely to lead to unhappiness for all parties.

One common example is to assume responsibility for "courtesy admissions," with the hospitalist admitting a physician's patient overnight and transferring patient care responsibility back to the physician the next day. Another example might involve hospitalists assisting with paperwork on patients they did not care for (e.g., expecting the hospitalist to do a discharge summary for a surgeon when the hospitalist was not involved in that patient's care).

The best strategy is to identify the most important services for the hospitalists to provide and initially keep the list relatively small (e.g., admit unassigned emergency medical patients, accept referrals from primary care physicians, and perform consults from other doctors). Other services can be added when hospitalist staffing allows (e.g., comanagement of some surgical admissions) and after the hospitalists have had an opportunity to participate in deciding which services are the most appropriate to add.

6. Allowing Excessive Workload, Leading to Hospitalist Dissatisfaction

A variety of factors can lead to excessive hospitalist workloads or patient volumes. The most common reason for an excessive workload is a referral volume that grows faster than staff can be added. In other cases hospitalists can make the mistake of scheduling each doctor to work relatively few days or shifts annually, resulting in a high workload for each day worked (even though the annual patient volume may not be excessive).

Hospitalists, like other professionals, seek balance in their job. The biggest threat to this goal is excessive workloads, which can hinder a hospitalist's ability to devote adequate attention to ensuring the satisfaction of patients and referring physicians. It also limits the hospitalist's ability to assume nonclinical responsibilities like protocol development and serving on hospital committees. Some data suggest that at some point an increasing patient load begins to result in an increasing length of stay (Hoxhaj, Hearne, and Bacon 2004). Over time, it is likely to result in poor job satisfaction, burnout, and turnover among physicians in the group.

7. Having Insufficient Financial Support

As mentioned in Chapter 4, SHM (2006) survey data indicate that 97 percent of hospitalist practices receive financial support and/or services in kind in addition to collected professional fees. This money usually comes from the hospital in which the hospitalists work.

Under some combination of the following conditions, hospitalist practices may require minimal or no subsidy funds:

- Hospitalists work only weekday hours.
- Hospitalists are not responsible for emergency, unassigned patients.
- Hospitalists have an excellent payer mix.

Otherwise, practices such as those that accept all emergency-department-unassigned medical admissions and/or have a hospitalist on-site 24/7 will have professional fee collections that fall far short of the amount needed to pay competitive salaries. As discussed in Chapter 4, these practices need outside financial support or must maintain high patient volumes to ensure enough revenue to pay reasonable salaries and benefits to the doctors. These practices are at risk of poor performance or collapse.

CONCLUSION

This chapter provided a high-level look at the key factors to building a successful hospitalist program and the key pitfalls that can lead to failure. If hospital executives and hospitalists work together to address these issues, they are likely to achieve some level of success with their hospitalists. Many topics raised in this chapter are covered in greater detail elsewhere in this book.

REFERENCES

Hoxhaj, S., L. Hearne, and A. Bacon. 2004. "Increasing Hospitalist Physician–Patient Ratios Leads to Decreased Efficiency." Abstract presented at the Society of Hospital Medicine Annual Meeting, New Orleans, LA, April 20.

Society of Hospital Medicine (SHM). 2006. *2005–2006 SHM Survey: State of the Hospital Medicine Movement.* Philadelphia, PA: Society of Hospital Medicine.

CHAPTER 6

Legal and Contract Issues in Hospitalist Practice

Key Message

Legal arrangements between a hospital and a hospital group must address relevant laws and regulations (e.g., Stark Law, antikickback statute, and gainsharing). Contracts must reflect the unique roles and responsibilities of hospitalists.

BACKGROUND

Hospitalists occupy a unique place on the healthcare landscape—at the intersection of the hospital's interests and those of the hospitalists themselves—both as a group and as individuals. The field of hospital medicine was spawned in part because of the need for hospitals and/or medical groups to manage hospital bed days and ancillary utilization as efficiently as possible. In the mid-1990s, research was published documenting that hospitalists often had lower lengths of stay and costs per case compared to traditional inpatient care (Wachter and Goldman 2002). This realization became a major driver of hospitalist growth.

Hospitalists were unable to make an adequate income from professional-fee revenues alone. They were motivated to negotiate with hospitals such that they (the hospitalists) could share in some of the hospital's cost savings engendered through lower costs per case (Polgrean 1997).

Hospitals were struggling to contain costs and lengths of stay under traditional inpatient care models. They were willing to consider new approaches to motivating physicians to control costs. Sharing cost savings with hospitalists would address this opportunity. Unfortunately, gainsharing arrangements, whereby hospitalists could receive monetary rewards proportionate to hospital cost savings, were rejected by a July 1999 ruling by the Office of Inspector General (OIG).

In the early 2000s, with the gainsharing prohibition and other limitations established by the Ethics in Patient Referrals Act (42 U.S.C. § 1395nn), commonly referred to as the Stark law, and the federal anti-kickback statute (42 U.S.C. § 1320a-7b.), it was not clear if and how hospitals and hospitalists would be able to partner and align incentives. However, hospitalist programs have flourished despite these obstacles. Most hospitals have been able to develop successful practices despite the constraints of these laws. Society of Hospital Medicine's *2005–2006 Productivity and Compensation Survey* found that 97 percent of hospital medicine groups receive financial support from either the hospital or from another sponsoring entity, such as a medical group (SHM 2006).

On the other hand, anecdotal observations support the notion that hospital administrators harbor concerns over the legality of arrangements that pay hospitalists for their services. These concerns may be affecting the availability of hospital financial support for hospitalist services.

This chapter is intended to provide an overview of legal and contracting issues in hospitalist practice and is in no way a substitute for expert legal counsel, which all parties should retain in any contracting process.

STARK LAW

The Stark law prohibits physicians from referring Medicare or Medicaid patients to an entity for the provision of what is known as "designated health services" if the physician (or an immediate family member) has a financial relationship with the entity. Under the law, a referral includes a physician sending a patient to a service provider (e.g., a laboratory) with which she has a financial relationship. In this context, a financial relationship refers to any ownership or investment interest or compensation arrangement with the entity, unless an exception applies.

The original intent of the Stark law pertained to physician-owned laboratories. Congress attempted to restrict the ability of physicians to refer to laboratories they owned to avoid overutilization of laboratory services. The current version of the law covers not only laboratory referrals but also a range of services, including physical therapy, imaging, durable medical equipment, prosthetic devices, and inpatient and outpatient hospital services (Knoll, in press). Lawmakers realized that a referral prohibition would be unworkable without some exceptions. When a physician complies with these exceptions, he may refer to a designated health services entity without violating the law.

How does the Stark law apply to hospitalists? If a hospitalist orders an imaging test at a facility with which he has any kind of financial relationship, then Stark law may be violated. To avoid such a violation, an exception must be invoked such as the "employment" or "personal services" exception outlined below (Knoll, in press):

- For employed hospitalists, the employment exception states that compensation for the employee—in this case, the ordering hospitalist—is set in advance, does not exceed fair market value, and is not determined in such a way that is dependent on volume or value of referrals in question.
- For contracted hospitalists, the personal services exception stipulates that (1) payment to the hospitalist must not be based on the volume or value of referrals by the hospitalist, (2) the agreement must be set out in writing, (3) the agreement must be a term of at least one year, and (4) compensation

must be set in advance. Other requirements also apply, which are beyond the scope of this chapter.

If a hospitalist is paid on an incentive that varies with, for example, reductions in length of stay or cost per case, the incentive violates the Stark law. If, on the other hand, the hospitalist is paid a set annual stipend under the title of director of inpatient services, then such an arrangement, if in compliance with the other elements of the personal services exception and other laws governing the relationship, is permissible. Compliance with Stark law is one of the most compelling reasons for close legal oversight of how hospital–hospitalist contracts are drawn up.

ANTIKICKBACK STATUTE

The antikickback statute makes it illegal for anyone to receive monies or other compensation for referring patients to a particular provider for services paid for by the Centers for Medicare & Medicaid Services (i.e., Medicare and Medicaid). The intent of antikickback legislation is to prevent the receipt of payments in exchange for referrals. Antikickback statutes apply to hospitalists in much the same way Stark law does: If a hospitalist refers a patient for a test or other service at the hospital at which she is employed or with whom she is contracted, contractual language will be needed that provides a safe harbor from the invocation of the antikickback statute. Fortunately, the safe harbor provisions for the antikickback law closely parallel those of the Stark law.

GAINSHARING

In a special advisory bulletin in July 1999, the OIG categorically prohibited hospitals from paying physicians a portion of cost savings that may have been a result of the effort of the physician

(OIG Special Advisory 1999). For hospitalists, this applies to cost savings resulting from shorter lengths of stay and reduced ancillary utilization. Since 1999, gainsharing has been reevaluated, and there have been several examples of approved gainsharing arrangements between physicians and hospitals. Each of these has involved medical/surgical devices or prostheses and therefore is not relevant to the case where hospitalists may share in savings resulting from reduced utilization of hospital resources. However, gainsharing remains an active topic in healthcare law, and Congress has approved several demonstration programs that allow experiments that may eventually have an impact on hospitalists.

CONTRACTING: HOSPITALIST EMPLOYMENT CONTRACTS

Employment contracts are agreements between a physician and an employing entity. To see a sample hospitalist employment contract, go to ache.org/books/Hospitalists. A list of the most important issues to consider in a hospitalist employment contract is contained in Figure 6.1. A number of issues are unique to hospitalists, especially those related to workload, work hours, schedule, and time off. Therefore, while including as many specifics as possible in an employment agreement is important, specifying all work conditions in the contract is not realistic and may be counterproductive.

Figure 6.1. Key Elements of Hospitalist Employment Contracts

- Employee vs. independent contractor
- Term, renewability, and termination
- Duties and responsibilities
- Compensation, incentives, and fringe benefits
- Credentialing
- Work schedule and time off
- Professional liability insurance and tail coverage
- Partnership track

Employee Versus Independent Contractor

Correctly classifying the hospitalist as an employee or independent contractor is an important step. Significant financial implications of classification as one or the other are at play, related to responsibility to pay employment tax, fringe benefits, and eligibility to participate in retirement plans. Also, certain exceptions to Stark Law vary depending on employee versus independent contractor status.

Term, Renewability, and Termination

The "term" defines the duration of a contract. Every contract should clearly state how long it will be in effect. "Renewability" pertains to the conditions for renewing the agreement. Some contracts automatically renew while others do not. Therefore, contracts should state conditions for renewal or if renewal is automatic. Finally, the contract must address the issue of its "termination." If the contract can only be terminated for cause, it is important to list the specific causes and the time period to remedy the identified cause. It is also important to specify the time period of advance written notice to end the agreement, regardless of whether cause exists.

Duties and Responsibilities

A hospitalist contract should provide a listing of clinical and non-clinical responsibilities and duties. Clinical duties require describing patient care activities, their location, and their scope. Nonclinical responsibilities include committee meetings, reporting requirements, and communication expectations. In the case of employees, it should be specified if moonlighting is permitted. Moonlighting is not uncommon for hospitalists, because they often work a nontraditional schedule and may have several consecutive days off, which can provide an opportunity to moonlight elsewhere. Many approaches to this issue are reasonable, and practices often allow moonlighting, if it is specifically approved by the practice director and if it does not interfere with the doctor's obligations to the parent practice. If prohibitions of non-income-generating activities are in place, such as lecturing or performing civic work, they should be specified.

Compensation, Incentives, and Fringe Benefits

The methods by which the hospitalist is compensated should be delineated in the agreement. If compensation is derived from a composite of base pay and incentives, this should be specified in detail. Factors that may affect base pay, such as number of annual hours worked over a target, should be precisely spelled out. The elements of an incentive scheme should be listed in a way that is comprehensible, such that the intended behavior on the part of the hospitalist may be fostered. In general, incentives that reward clinical productivity (billing) and quality of care are permissible. Incentives that promote utilization efficiency, such as reductions in length of stay or cost per case, are not permissible under Stark law and gainsharing prohibitions. A complete listing of employee benefits should be provided.

Credentialing

Requirements for training and certification should be listed.

Work Schedule and Time Off

Scheduling is a difficult and potentially confusing topic in hospitalist contracting because hospitalists must cover a 24/7/365-day schedule that does not fit neatly into a traditional weekday-weekend-holiday paradigm. Also, because most hospitalist programs are growing and have changing work demands, the ability to specify a fixed schedule over time is nearly impossible.

One challenge in a contract is establishing the definition of a full-time equivalent (FTE) hospitalist.

- For many hospitalists it is best to use annual hours to define an FTE. This approach is often used where hospitalists are employees (of hospitals or medical schools) and expect to have clearly defined work expectations.
  o Note: If a weekly hour amount is needed, derive this from the annual hours, adjusted for specified vacation time. For example, if 1,932 annual hours define an FTE and the contract specifies four weeks of vacation and two weeks of education time, then the number of work hours in a week can be stated as 1,932/46 = 42.
- When a substantial portion of a hospitalist's compensation is based on production, it may not be necessary to define an FTE hospitalist in terms of annual hours. In these situations, hospitalists receive significant rewards for additional work. It may make more sense to simply hire a physician as a member of the group and for the group to then determine a fair and equitable way to distribute the work. This approach may be more common for hospitalists who are part of a private group (i.e., a local or national hospitalist group or a multispecialty group).

A related issue is whether a contract should specify vacation, time off for continuing medical education (CME), and other time off.

- If vacation and other time off are specified in the contract, the following should be avoided:
  o Specifying in a contract which days (e.g., holidays) or weeks a hospitalist may take off (This should be worked out by the group.)
  o Putting into a contract a fixed schedule with specified shifts

o Specifying in a contract the frequency of off hours worked (e.g., weekends or nights)
- However, an alternative approach is to simply specify the amount of work required from the hospitalist (e.g., x hours annually). Any nonworking time can be used for vacation, CME time, or some other category of time off.

Professional Liability Insurance and Tail Coverage

Details of professional liability insurance, including the carrier and type (occurrence or claims made) should be stated. In an employer–employee arrangement, the party paying for the insurance should be delineated, as should the party bearing responsibility for paying tail coverage for claims-made policies. Independent contractors usually pay for their own malpractice insurance, unless otherwise stated.

In some instances, a departing doctor's tail coverage is paid by the practice only if he leaves after a short period of employment (e.g., two years or less). After that point, the doctor would become responsible for paying for his own tail coverage. This approach may be problematic for hospitalists. Hospitalist practice has relatively low barriers to entry and exit for a doctor, and hospitalists often consider changing jobs or careers every few years. Cases can be cited where hospitalists were reasonably content with their practice, but when faced with the responsibility for paying their own tail coverage (e.g., by staying beyond the second year of employment) they leave the practice to avoid this risk. For this reason many practices, especially those in which hospitals employ hospitalists, have decided that the employer will pay the tail coverage regardless of the doctor's duration of employment.

Partnership Track

For private groups that are not hospital employed, often an option to become a partner or owner of the hospitalist group is offered. In this case, the employment contract should provide the conditions for achieving partnership status, including how long before eligibility and the terms for partner status. The implications of partner status, such as the ability to influence group decisions, sharing in group revenues, and exposure to group liability, should be fully understood.

It is important for each hospitalist group to think carefully about the rationale for a partnership track. Hospitalist groups may be different from other forms of physician practice in that the practice itself may have little or no market value. Becoming a partner may not be associated with an increase in the value of an asset. Instead, partnership for a hospitalist might simply mean obtaining a vote in group decisions and/or an increase in compensation.

CONTRACTING: PROFESSIONAL SERVICES CONTRACTS

Professional services contracts are agreements between a hospitalist group and a third party, such as a hospital, payer, or physician organization (e.g., an independent practice association). Similar to hospitalist employment contracts, these agreements may specify the hospitalist group as either an employee or an independent contractor. The elements listed under the preceding employment contracts section also apply in professional services contracts. In addition, the following elements warrant special consideration in a professional services contract:

- Covered services and terms of the contract
- Compensation and incentives
- Utilization management and other support services

Covered Services and Terms of the Contract

"Covered services" refers to the scope of services defined by the agreement. It includes clinical responsibilities and administrative elements. Clinical elements include the following:

- *Patient age and type.* Examples are uninsured patients requiring admission through the emergency department (ED), insured patients with no primary physician requiring admission, and patients who are older than age 17 with a medical diagnosis.
- *Facilities and units.* This specifies which hospitals and units are covered—for example, the ED (for triage purposes), skilled nursing or rehabilitation units, and so forth.

Administrative elements include the following:

- *Reporting requirements.* These include quality, efficiency, or satisfaction metrics. Sample metrics might include readmission rates, avoidable bed days, adverse events, primary physician satisfaction, ED response times, and length of stay. Frequency and modality (e.g., electronic or paper) of reporting may be specified.
- *Meetings.* These include meetings of the joint (referring to representatives from both contract parties) operating committee, utilization review committee, and discharge planning committee.

Compensation and Incentives

Compensation in a hospitalist contract depends on whether it is with a payer, such as a managed care organization (MCO), or a hospital. MCOs may pay hospitalists on a fee-for-service basis, using a case rate, or in a prepaid fashion through a capitated payment. Hospitals usually provide compensation to a hospitalist group through a fixed payment made at a predetermined interval. In the case of incentives provided either by a hospital or an MCO, generally those that reward enhanced quality of care or stakeholder satisfaction—such as primary physician or patient—are permissible. Incentives rewarding enhanced efficiency, such as reduced length of stay, reduced admission rates, or reduced cost per case, should be avoided because of the prohibitions under the

Stark law, antikickback statutes, and concerns over professional liability exposure.

Utilization Management and Other Support Services

MCO contracts should specify which party is responsible for utilization management, including (1) the method and frequency of measuring utilization, (2) who is responsible for performing the utilization review activities, and (3) how utilization is reported. For hospital–hospitalist group contracts, support services provided by the hospital should be specified. Major categories include billing services, clerical support, case management/discharge planning, and information technology services for obtaining hospital quality, utilization, and satisfaction data. Also, office space, computers, furniture, white coats, and so forth provided by the hospital should be specified.

ANTITRUST LAW

Antitrust law is designed to facilitate competition in a free market for the benefit of consumers. In healthcare, three major clauses in professional services agreements, which on their face appear anticompetitive, are permissible by law. These are exclusivity clauses, restrictive covenants, and sweeps clauses. Table 6.1 describes each clause in detail.

CONCLUSION

This chapter has reviewed a number of laws that govern the rules by which hospitalists may contract with hospitals and other employing entities. The existence of statutes like the Stark law and the gainsharing prohibition should not deter hospitals and hospitalists from engaging in mutually beneficial arrangements, even

Table 6.1. Permissible Contract Clauses Under Antitrust Law

	Description	*Applicability to Hospitalists*
Exclusivity clauses	Contract granting the sole right to one group for provision of hospitalist services at an institution	• More difficult to apply to hospitalists than other hospital-based specialties because of difficulty in defining a "hospitalist" arrangement • May be applicable to specific service lines such as ED unassigned or medical care on rehabilitation unit
Restrictive covenants	Restrict how long and how far away a former hospitalist employee may compete with employer	• Not as valuable for hospitalists as for specialties, where patients may "follow" a physician to a competitor hospital • May hinder recruiting candidates because of restrictiveness, but may mitigate hospitalist turnover to local competitor groups
Sweeps clauses	Provision whereby hospital privileges for hospitalists are terminated if their group's contract is terminated	• Applies when a hospitalist group contract is terminated with an institution • Treated as a voluntary resignation; not reportable because no quality issue is involved

Source: Adapted from Knoll (in press). Used with permission.

if hospitals directly compensate the hospitalists for the value they provide.

The chapter has also provided an overview of important considerations in hospitalist employment and professional services agreements. While this resource may familiarize one with key issues in contracting, it is essential for all parties involved in negotiating a contract to retain diligent, qualified counsel to have their interests represented as effectively as possible.

REFERENCES

Knoll, A. In press. "Legal Issues in Hospital-Hospitalist Relationships." In *Comprehensive Hospital Medicine*, edited by M. V. Williams. Philadelphia, PA: Saunders.

Office of Inspector General (OIG) Special Advisory. 1999. "Gainsharing Arrangements and CMPs for Hospital Payments to Physicians to Reduce or Limit Services to Beneficiaries." [Online opinion; retrieved 2/17/07.] http://oig.hhs.gov/fraud/alertsandbulletins/gainsh.htm.

Polgrean, J. S. 1997. "Anti-Kickback Laws and Hospitalists: Is There Any Recourse?" *The Hospitalist* 1 (3): 3–8.

Society of Hospital Medicine (SHM). 2006. *2005–2006 Productivity and Compensation Survey.* Philadelphia, PA: Society of Hospital Medicine.

Wachter, R. M., and L. Goldman. 2002. "The Hospitalist Movement Five Years Later." *Journal of the American Medical Association* 287: (4) 487–94.

ADDITIONAL READINGS

Nelson, J. 2007. "The Vacation Conundrum." *The Hospitalist* 11 (3): 89, 91.

———. 2007. "Contractual Cautions: 2 Provisions That Require Careful Consideration." *The Hospitalist* 11 (4): 89, 91.

SECTION II

HOSPITAL MEDICINE: A PRACTICE MANAGEMENT PERSPECTIVE

CHAPTER 7

Hospitalist Retention and Career Satisfaction

Key Message

To address hospitalist retention and career satisfaction, four issues should be considered: reward/recognition, workload/schedule, autonomy/control, and community/environment.

With the advent of hospital medicine as a bona fide career track for physicians and the explosive growth of the specialty, the issue of career satisfaction and how best to retain qualified hospitalists has emerged as a challenge for hospitals and their hospital medicine groups. The complexity and uniqueness of each hospital's environment and the costs (financial and otherwise) of hospitalist turnover raise the value of having a stable group of hospitalists who are dedicated to their career, to the hospital medicine group, and to the institution.

THE SCOPE OF THE PROBLEM

Survey research quantifies the issues of hospitalist retention, burnout, and career satisfaction as follows:

- In 2005, the mean annual turnover rate for hospital medicine groups was 12 percent; 37 percent of groups had an annual turnover rate of 15 percent or greater (SHM 2006).
- In 2001, the reported burnout rate among hospitalists was 13 percent; an additional 25 percent of hospitalists were at risk for burnout (Hoff et al. 2001).
- In 2005, six of the top ten concerns of hospitalist group leaders related to career satisfaction: work hours and work–life balance, recruitment, expectations and demands from the hospital, professional respect and job satisfaction, career sustainability, and retention (SHM 2006) (see Figure 7.1).

No comparable data are available from other specialties; however, these figures clearly point to an important issue for the specialty of hospital medicine.

MAJOR AREAS AFFECTING HOSPITALIST RETENTION AND CAREER SATISFACTION

Hoff, Whitcomb, and Nelson (2002) investigated factors associated with hospitalist burnout and identified three major areas:

Figure 7.1. Top Concerns Identified by Hospitalist Group Leaders

- Work hours/work–life balance—42%
- Recruitment—35%
- Daily workload—29%
- Expectations/demands from hospital—23%
- Reimbursement/collections—17%
- Professional respect/job satisfaction—17%
- Career sustainability—15%
- Retention—15%
- Quality of care/quality indicators—13%
- Specialist availability for consultation—11%
- Bed capacity/throughput—11%
- Scheduling—11%

Note: Each survey respondent was asked to choose three concerns. The responses reflect the proportion of respondents selecting each option.

Source: SHM (2006).

---

1. Perceived lack of autonomy
2. Poor recognition by patients and families
3. Lack of occupational solidarity (not feeling part of a close-knit group of peer professionals)

More recently, Society of Hospital Medicine (SHM) chartered the Career Satisfaction Task Force to research the topic and make recommendations. The task force prepared a white paper, which developed the framework depicted in Figure 7.2 (Career Satisfaction Task Force 2006).

For individual hospitalists, the task force's framework is concerned with job fit based on four areas of job control that contribute to career satisfaction:

Figure 7.2. A Framework for Hospitalist Career Satisfaction

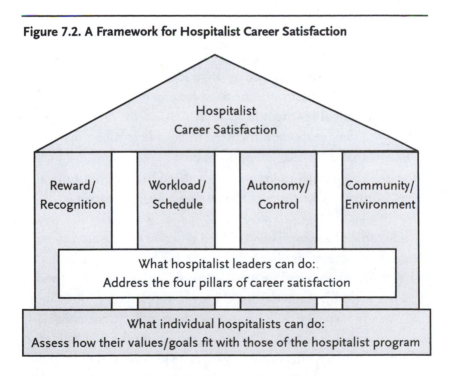

Source: Career Satisfaction Task Force (2006).

1. *Task control:* control over when, how, and how quickly a task is done
2. *Decision/organizational control:* control over task assignment and policies
3. *Physical environment control:* control over the location, layout, and climate of where work is done
4. *Resource control:* control over the availability of support staff, supplies, and materials

SHM developed a questionnaire (see Figure 7.3) that helps hospitalists understand their personal priorities and values with regard to job control and evaluate these control elements in their current and potential work situation.

With regard to areas that hospitalist leaders can influence, the task force's framework addresses four topics, depicted as the four pillars in the diagram:

Pillar 1—Reward/recognition: the need for appropriate reward—monetary and nonmonetary—for a job well done
Pillar 2—Workload/schedule: the need for a manageable workload and a sustainable schedule
Pillar 3—Autonomy/control: the need to be able to affect the key factors that influence job performance
Pillar 4—Community/environment: the need for a community and environment that support a satisfying, engaging career

The topic of appropriate workload deserves special attention, as it can be an issue of conflict between the hospital and the hospitalists. A business case can be made for keeping the workload manageable for hospitalists. Hoxhaj, Hearne, and Bacon (2004) show that once the average daily census per hospitalist went above 14, length of stay rose sharply. Therefore, subjecting the hospitalists to inordinately heavy workloads may increase lengths of stay and costs under a diagnosis-related group payment system. The result will be avoidable expense on the hospital side of the balance sheet that is

Figure 7.3. Job-Fit Questionnaire—Sample Questions

INSTRUCTIONS: Assess your perceived control and its importance on each of the following items. Please circle your response. Note two scales for each item: the top scale indicates amount of control you currently have, and the bottom scale represents the amount of desire for control. Identify the gaps between having control and wanting control.

Amount of Control You Currently Have	Amount of Desire for Control
1 = no control over item 2 = minimal control over item 3 = some control over item 4 = significant control over item 5 = total control over item	1 = not important at all to have control over item 2 = slightly important to have control over item 3 = desire some control over item 4 = desire significant control over item 5 = absolutely must have control over item

Task

Set the pace of work   Amount of control you currently have   1 2 3 4 5
                       Amount of desire for control   1 2 3 4 5

Decision

Select consultants   Amount of control you currently have   1 2 3 4 5
                     Amount of desire for control   1 2 3 4 5

Influence/change   Amount of control you currently have   1 2 3 4 5
hospital policy   Amount of desire for control   1 2 3 4 5

Environment

Which nursing unit   Amount of control you currently have   1 2 3 4 5
you work on   Amount of desire for control   1 2 3 4 5

Resources

Computer terminal   Amount of control you currently have   1 2 3 4 5
availability   Amount of desire for control   1 2 3 4 5

Source: Society of Hospital Medicine, Philadelphia, PA.

likely to exceed any added professional-fee revenues for the hospital medicine group. This analysis did not take into account other costs, specifically:

- Lost throughput opportunity associated with longer lengths of stay (i.e., new patients might have to be turned away)
- The cost of physician turnover resulting from burnout

CAREER SATISFACTION FOR HOSPITALISTS: WHAT CAN BE DONE?

SHM's white paper on career satisfaction outlines five categories of action steps (Career Satisfaction Task Force 2006):

1. *Get the facts:* information from research, analyses, and/or surveys that can help address particular career satisfaction issues
2. *Organizational/structural strategies:* formal steps that can be taken with regard to the structure of the hospitalist group, how it is staffed, and/or how hospitalists are compensated
3. *Systems strategies:* changes that can be made to the operation (processes) of the hospitalist group
4. *Professional development strategies:* actions that can be taken directed at individual hospitalists
5. *Marketing/relationship strategies:* how hospitalists can redefine how they relate to other key stakeholders in their work environment

A summary of suggested action steps in these five categories for each of the four pillars is presented in Appendix D. In addition, the white paper recommends some "fundamental concepts"—the basics and leadership principles—that serve to both integrate and enhance the ideas in the framework. These are described in the following sections.

The Basics

- Recognize each hospitalist as an individual. Each hospitalist has his own preferences, interests, and goals.
- Ensure that adequate environmental resources are in place. Before the more sophisticated satisfaction issues can be addressed, sufficient administrative support, space, and equipment must be in place.
- Ensure that adequate professional development support is available in the form of peer groups or individual supervision and mentoring.
- Make informed decisions. Addressing hospitalist career satisfaction requires making sure that all parties understand the current state of affairs and the available options.

Leadership Principles

- Build a cohesive team. Individual hospitalists will be more satisfied when they feel like they are part of a group with similar values, philosophies, and attitudes.
- Build positive relationships. The hospitalist practice does not operate in a vacuum. Addressing career satisfaction requires positive relationships with hospital leadership, members of the medical staff, and nonphysician healthcare professionals.
- Create an ownership mentality. If hospitalists are to be treated with respect, they must view their group in a manner similar to private physicians in the community. This includes having a shared sense of accountability for the practice's performance, including financial matters.
- Operate the practice in a businesslike manner. There should be some formality to the hospitalist practice (e.g., a business plan, negotiated service agreements, and annual budgets).

CONCLUSION

With the growth of the hospital medicine specialty and the tight job market, recruiting and retaining quality hospitalists are critical, high-priority issues. Hospital executives and hospitalists themselves will need to work together to address the risks of career dissatisfaction and burnout.

REFERENCES

Career Satisfaction Task Force. 2006. "A Challenge for a New Specialty: A White Paper on Hospitalist Career Satisfaction." Philadelphia, PA: Society of Hospital Medicine.

Hoff, T. J., W. F. Whitcomb, K. Williams, J. R. Nelson, and R. A. Cheesman. 2001. "Characteristics and Work Experiences of Hospitalists in the United States." *Archives of Internal Medicine* 161 (6): 851–58.

Hoff, T., W. F. Whitcomb, and J. R. Nelson. 2002. "Thriving and Surviving in a New Medical Career: The Case of Hospitalist Physicians." *Journal of Health and Social Behavior* 43 (March): 72–91.

Hoxhaj, S., L. Hearne, and A. Bacon. 2004. "Increasing Hospitalist Physician-Patient Ratios Lead to Decreased Hospital Efficiency." Abstract presented to the Society of Hospital Medicine Annual Meeting, New Orleans, LA, April 19–21.

Society of Hospital Medicine (SHM). 2006. *2005–2006 SHM Survey: State of the Hospital Medicine Movement.* Philadelphia, PA: Society of Hospital Medicine.

CHAPTER 8

Use of Nonphysician Clinical Staff in Hospitalist Programs

Key Message

Consider the following issues before incorporating physician assistants (PAs) and/or nurse practitioners (NPs) into a hospital medicine group:

- Do the physician hospitalists in the group buy into the PA/NP paradigm?
- Is the group stable enough to support the incorporation of PAs/NPs?
- Is there an understanding on how to bill for PA/NP services?
- Are qualified PA/NP candidates available?

The hospital is perhaps the ideal setting for collaborative relationships among healthcare professionals. As hospital executives are aware, effective patient care in a modern hospital requires close working relationships among a variety of professional disciplines. It is in this context that the use of nonphysician clinical staff began to flourish within hospital medicine programs. This chapter describes the various nonphysician staff who work closely and directly with physician hospitalists in clinical matters. These professionals may be categorized as follows:

- Physician assistants (PAs)
- Nurse practitioners (NPs)
- Care managers and coordinators
- Rounding assistants

The role of nonclinical support personnel, such as the hospital medicine practice manager, and others will not be discussed in this chapter.

NURSE PRACTITIONERS AND PHYSICIAN ASSISTANTS

In recent years, the growth in the number of PAs and NPs functioning as part of a hospitalist team has been substantial. Fueled by a demand for hospitalists that exceeds the supply and the fact that their compensation is less than that of physicians, in 2005 PAs and NPs could be found in 16 percent and 20 percent, respectively, of hospital medicine groups (SHM 2006). Parallel with this growth is a burgeoning body of literature supporting the value of these professionals in the care of hospitalized patients, often the critically ill (Rudy et al. 1998; Hoffman et al. 2005; Cowan et al. 2006). While differences exist in the training and the care provided by PAs versus NPs, for the purposes of this discussion, the two will be considered together.

In 2004, Society of Hospital Medicine issued a policy statement delineating the conditions under which PAs and NPs should be incorporated into a hospital medicine practice, offering a supportive view of the role of these professionals as hospitalists. Yet despite broad support, robust growth in numbers, and increasing evidence supporting their use, a wide range of PA/NP work models are seen in hospitalist groups. No clear consensus has been achieved on the best way to use PAs and NPs as a physician adjunct while avoiding pitfalls inherent in nonphysicians caring for complex, acutely ill hospitalized patients (Ottley,

Agbontaen, and Wilkow 2000). Some guidance on this topic is presented in the following sections.

What Do PA/NP Hospitalists Do?

In the best sense, a PA/NP extends the clinical reach of the physician. This means that the PA/NP performs many of the tasks of a physician, with the difference being that a supervisory relationship exists such that the physician oversees the clinical activity of the PA/NP. Society of Hospital Medicine (2006) queried group leaders who employ PAs or NPs about the activities of the PAs/NPs in their group (the respondents were instructed to choose the top five activities). The results, shown below, describe the most common roles of PAs/NPs:

- Perform patient rounds: 83 percent
- Write prescriptions: 82 percent
- Take histories and perform physicals: 77 percent
- Communicate with primary care physicians: 72 percent
- Act as an initial responder: 66 percent
- Participate in discharge planning: 66 percent

Figure 8.1 provides a more comprehensive list of PA/NP responsibilities, for the purposes of understanding their scope of practice in hospital medicine and developing job descriptions.

Factors to Consider Before Bringing in PAs/NPs

A number of factors must be considered before deciding to incorporate PAs or NPs into a hospital medicine group. Because of the complexity of hospitalized patient care, some physician hospitalists may be reluctant to work with them. Obtaining hospitalist group buy-in is essential to the successful long-term incorporation of PAs

Figure 8.1. Potential Clinical Responsibilities of PA/NP Hospitalists

- Coordinate patient admissions, including data gathering, order writing, and attending to urgent patients pending physician arrival.
- Coordinate discharge activities, including preparation of discharge summaries, patient education, discharge planning, and care coordination.
- Take histories, and perform physical examinations.
- Diagnose and manage acute and chronic health conditions according to the best available evidence.
- Order and interpret diagnostic studies and laboratory tests.
- Perform appropriate diagnostic and therapeutic procedures, including central-line placement and lumbar puncture.
- Prescribe pharmacologic therapies, including controlled medications.
- Consult appropriate specialists for patient care needs.
- Assist patients in coping with illness.
- Perform consultation and follow-up on surgical patients.
- Communicate patient status in a timely fashion with referring physician, including at admission, discharge, and other times as appropriate.
- Work with committees to improve systems and processes of care.
- Assist with documentation of relevant billing information and development of efficient billing processes.

or NPs. Also, the hospital medicine group must be stable. A chaotic hospital medicine group with turnover, poor leadership, or a general lack of focus regarding the group's mission will create barriers to fostering close ties between the PAs/NPs and the physicians. Of course, appropriate billing practices must be in place and well understood when using PAs/NPs, and qualified candidates must be available for the position.

The effective deployment of PAs and NPs as hospitalists requires planning to prevent their misuse (such as caring for excessively ill or complex patients without adequate supervision) or their ineffective use (such as physician duplication of the PA's or NP's work, thereby negating the value of the PA/NP as a physician extender). One strategy that may be particularly effective is to place the PA/NP on a single unit, such as an acute rehabilitation or neurology unit, to create a sense of ownership and control over the work performed.

It is crucial to limit the number of physician work relationships for a PA/NP, especially an inexperienced one. The effective PA/NP forms a bond with a few physicians, from whom she learns and develops a functional working relationship. Setting aside structured time each day to review patient care issues is necessary for an appropriate level of supervision. Finally, measures must be taken to minimize the perception on the part of the medical staff and patients that a PA/NP is but one more factor in the fragmentation of care among many providers. Table 8.1 lists approaches to embrace and avoid when using PA/NP hospitalists.

Specific Approaches to Successfully Using PAs and NPs

Integrating PAs/NPs into a hospital medicine practice is a major challenge. A principled, thoughtful approach is essential to achieving good patient outcomes and a meaningful, positive experience for the PA/NP and supervising physician. Table 8.2 provides three models for successfully using PAs/NPs: first responder, unit-based provider, and traditional hospitalist.

Regulatory and Oversight Issues

Procedures for PA/NP billing, the legality of writing prescriptions, and physician oversight requirements vary from state to state. Prior to incorporating PAs or NPs into a hospital medicine practice, it is essential to establish policies covering these areas that are compliant with state law. It is advisable to work with the practice's billing service to ensure compliance with accepted billing practices and to educate the overseeing physician(s) regarding their responsibilities. State boards of registration in medicine have policy statements addressing these areas,

Table 8.1. Dos and Don'ts in Working with PA/NP Hospitalists

Do	Don't
Pair the PA/NP with one or two mentor hospitalists, especially in the first several months, to form a strong working relationship and trust in each other's clinical abilities.	Have the PA/NP, especially an inexperienced one, work with several hospitalists. The PA/NP can be overwhelmed with multiple practice styles and fail to form vital professional bonds with a small number of physician hospitalists.
Set aside dedicated time in the day to distribute work and to review specific patient care issues.	Assume that a casual approach to work distribution and review of patient management with the PA/NP will suffice. Often, the PA/NP will be under- or unsupervised, exposing quality and regulatory gaps.
Ensure that regular educational forums are scheduled, where evidence-based and best practices are reviewed.	Neglect to provide physician education to the PA/NP on a regular basis, especially in the course of patient care.
For the PA/NP's patients, ensure that the physician hospitalist maintains a strong presence when communicating with patients, families, and referring physicians.	Give the impression to patients, families, and referring physicians that the PA/NP is managing patient care with lax supervision. Referring physicians do not want to send their acutely ill patients to someone with less training.
Create tasks and a work flow that challenge the PAs/NPs but do not overwhelm them.	Assign PAs/NPs tasks that they are overqualified to perform, such as collecting x-rays or clinical data or doing clinical secretarial work. PAs and NPs have been trained to provide patient care and should be employed in this capacity.
Create a group culture where the PAs/NPs feel valued and where their concerns can be legitimately heard.	Treat the PAs/NPs as if they have little say in group decisions simply because they are not as highly trained as the physician hospitalist.

Table 8.2. Three Models for the Successful Use of PA/NP Hospitalists

Role	Responsibility
First responder to patients requiring admission or urgent/emergent patients	• Provide timely history and physical and treatment plans for patients in the emergency department or patients who have been directly admitted to the hospital • Work with rapid response team, code blue team, or physician hospitalists to rapidly assess potentially unstable patients until additional resources arrive • Schedule: Days, evenings, and/or overnights
Unit-based provider	• Staff a single unit (e.g., acute rehabilitation, psychiatry, telemetry, intensive care unit) • Provide direct patient care in conjunction with a supervising physician hospitalist • Serve as the hospitalist representative to unit-based multidisciplinary team; attend team meetings and be available for less formal interaction with members of the team • Schedule: Typically a traditional daytime schedule, with occasional weekend duties
Traditional hospitalist	• Provide admission histories and physicals; develop treatment plans • Perform daily patient rounds • Coordinate discharges • Work with multidisciplinary team on individual patient care issues • Work with multidisciplinary team to improve systems, quality, patient safety, efficiency, and stakeholder satisfaction • Schedule: Most effective when scheduled alongside a single physician hospitalist or a small number of physician hospitalists

and the professional societies for PAs and NPs are good sources of information. The hospital's bylaws should be consulted in the early stages of incorporating PAs and NPs into the practice to ensure compliance.

CARE MANAGERS AND COORDINATORS

Care managers (often referred to as case managers or clinical care coordinators) are an essential component of hospitalist efficiency. The foundation of an effective care manager–hospitalist relationship is a structured communication system whereby real-time information is passed between the two regarding any issue related to patient disposition and discharge planning. In some instances, hospitalists and care managers participate in a formal meeting each day in which patient status is discussed.

ROUNDING ASSISTANTS

A growing number of hospital medicine programs are incorporating professionals who assist hospitalists in the course of daily work in much the same way an office nurse or medical assistant may support a physician with an office practice. Often referred to as a rounding assistant, this individual performs tasks that can improve the efficiency of the hospitalist. Rounding assistants typically do not require training beyond that of a medical assistant. The rounding assistant may be responsible for the following:

- Gathering clinical data, such as selected elements of patient history, medication list, allergies, past medical and surgical history, and vaccination status
- Obtaining information from referring physicians, nursing homes, and prior hospitals
- Assembling hospitalist data for daily rounding, such as patient vital signs; intake/output; blood glucose readings; stool guaiacs;

updated medication list; and objective data, including laboratory, radiology, microbiology, and pathology results

- Notifying referring physician when patient is admitted, discharged, or transferred
- Assisting hospitalist with family/loved one communication
and status updates
- Conveying patient information to discharge planning staff to
facilitate patient flow
- Facilitating transfer of information to the accepting physician
and venue of care at the time of discharge
- Assisting hospitalist with the professional-fee billing process,
including capture of Current Procedural Terminology and
ICD-10 diagnoses, patient demographic and insurance data,
and evaluation and management of billing information

CONCLUSION

The use of nonphysicians in collaboration with physician hospitalists
can contribute to the quality and efficiency of care for hospitalized
patients. Indeed it is only within the context of the broader hospital
team that a physician can be truly effective. To realize the potential and
avoid pitfalls that may be encountered, a carefully considered approach
is required. This overview is intended to provide guidance in both the
planning and execution stages of using nonphysician staff so that an
optimal return on this investment is realized.

REFERENCES

Cowan, M. J., M. Shapiro, R. D. Hays, A. Afifi, S. Vazirani, and S. L. Ettner. 2006. "The
Effect of a Multidisciplinary, Hospitalist/Physician and Advanced Practice Nurse
Collaboration on Hospital Costs." *Journal of Nursing Administration* 36 (2): 79–85.

Hoffman, L., F. Tasota, T. G. Zullo, C. Scharfenberg, and M. P. Donahoe. 2005.
"Outcomes of Care Managed by an Acute Care Nurse Practitioner/Attending

Physician Team in a Subacute Medical Intensive Care Unit." *American Journal of Critical Care* 14 (March): 121–30.

Ottley, R., J. X. Agbontaen, and B. R. Wilkow. 2000. "The Hospitalist PA: An Emerging Opportunity." *Journal of the American Academy of Physician Assistants* 13 (11): 21–28.

Rudy, E. B., L. J. Davidson, B. Daly, J. M. Clochesy, S. Sereika, M. Baldisseri, M. Hravnak, T. Ross, and C. Ryan. 1998. "Care Activities and Outcomes of Patients Cared for by Acute Care Nurse Practitioners, Physician Assistants, and Resident Physicians: A Comparison." *American Journal of Critical Care* 7: 267–81.

Society of Hospital Medicine (SHM). 2004. "SHM Policy Statement on Physician Assistants and Nurse Practitioners in Hospital Medicine." [Online policy statement; retrieved 02/22/07.] www.hospitalmedicine.org.

———. 2006. *2005–2006 SHM Survey: State of the Hospital Medicine Movement.* Philadelphia, PA: Society of Hospital Medicine.

CHAPTER 9

Communication in Hospitalist Programs

Key Message

The introduction of a hospitalist into the inpatient environment creates new communication challenges with patients, members of the medical staff, nurses, and other healthcare professionals.

The hospitalist model introduces a new player into the patient care process. Unlike the traditional model where one physician manages the patient in all settings, handoffs occur between a referring physician and a hospitalist on admission and discharge. This built-in discontinuity places a premium on the ability of members of the hospital team to transfer important information and communicate effectively with patients, family, nonhospital providers, and each other. Hospital executives should be aware that optimal communication in a hospital medicine program will require an investment in infrastructure.

The purpose of this chapter is to describe the scope of the communication issue and the resources required to support a successful hospital medicine program. This chapter focuses on the following key areas in communication:

- Between the hospitalist and the referring (or other involved) physicians
- Between the hospitalist and patients, family, and significant others
- Between the hospital leadership and the hospital medicine group

A sample communication plan for a hospital medicine group is presented in Appendix E.

COMMUNICATION WITH REFERRING PHYSICIANS

The research on communication between hospitalists and referring physicians indicates that certain risks are associated with patient transfers, that hospitalists are concerned about these risks, and that consensus has been reached on what information should be transmitted and when it should be transmitted (see Table 9.1).

In practice, determining the timing and content of communication is perhaps best left to the involved physicians, bearing in mind that the Joint Commission's (2007) *National Patient Safety Goals* mandate where organizations and providers must "implement a standardized approach to 'handoff' communications, including an opportunity to ask and respond to questions."

The Hospitalist's Role

The hospitalist plays a major role in ensuring that needed information is transmitted to the referring physician in prompt fashion. Responsibilities of the hospitalist include the following:

- Dictating history and physical (H&P) and discharge summary documents at the time of the patient encounter

Table 9.1. Research Findings: Hospitalist Communications

Study	Findings
Australian study of 350 general practitioners (Isaac et al. 1997) *Note:* Australia has long separated inpatient care and outpatient care	• 84% were not notified of their patient's hospital admission • 87% were not notified of major changes in their patient's condition • 75% were not notified of their patient's hospital discharge
Survey of U.S. hospitalists (Lindenauer et al. 1999)	Does the transition suffer from the handoff? • 8% regularly, 79% occasionally, 12% never When do you communicate with the primary care physician? • 93% at discharge, 82% at time of patient death, 75% on admission, 13% for daily progress, 10% for new test/medicine
Study of U.S. primary care physicians who refer to hospitalists (Pantilat et al. 2001)	When is it "very important" for hospitalists to communicate? • 73% on admission, 78% at discharge, 54% upon major patient-status change, 50% prior to major intervention What information is "very important" for hospitalists to communicate? • 94% discharge medications, 93% discharge diagnosis, 80% scheduled follow-up with primary care physician, 73% lab test results

- Ensuring that communication systems with referring physicians are operational and reliable
- When appropriate, making a phone call to the referring physician regarding admission/discharge and important events
- Informing the referring physician that a patient is admitted

and discharged, if H&Ps and discharge summaries are not available to that physician within a few hours of dictation

The Referring Physician's Role

An often overlooked element of communication is the role of the referring physician in ensuring that pertinent patient information is sent to the hospitalist. In a well-functioning hospital medicine program, the referring physician is an equal partner in the communication and transfer of information. The referring physician's office staff should have a mechanism in place to transmit pertinent office records to the hospitalist when a patient is admitted to the hospital. Some practices set up a system such that upon receipt of the hospitalist's H&P, the referring physician's clerical staff will automatically send pertinent office records to the hospital.

COMMUNICATION WITH PATIENTS, FAMILY, AND SIGNIFICANT OTHERS

The Hospitalist's Role

Communication with patients and loved ones is a core skill for hospitalists and one that carries high stakes because of the lack of a prior relationship with the patient. The hospitalist must communicate the following to patients:

- The nature of the referring physician–hospitalist collaboration (i.e., how the two communicate, how they coordinate care between inpatient and outpatient settings, how each furnishes the other with pertinent information)
- Expectations regarding hospitalist daily visits and availability for family meetings

- Hospitalist status updates and timely discussion of test results and management decisions
- How the discharge planning process works

It is important to distribute the hospitalist brochure at the outset of hospitalization to reinforce verbal communication. See Figure 9.1 for the key components of a hospital medicine group brochure and Appendix C for a sample brochure.

After discharge, an opportunity remains for communication with patients (Nelson 2001). This is a time when patients may not be clear on instructions, medications, and medical follow-up. A phone call to the patient by a hospitalist or other member of the hospital team soon after discharge may improve patient compliance with the treatment plan and other outcomes (Dudas et al. 2001).

The Referring Physician's Role

A potential pitfall is the feeling of abandonment some patients feel when "their doctor" (i.e., their primary care physician) seems to disappear from the care team during the episode of hospitalization. Often, the sense of abandonment can be averted by having the referring physician apprise the patient of the nature of her

---

Figure 9.1. Key Components of a Hospital Medicine Group Brochure

- Name, photograph, and short biographical sketch for each hospitalist
- Information on how to contact the hospitalist
- The relationship between the hospitalist and the referring physician, including how the two communicate
- Why the patient is under the care of a hospitalist instead of his personal physician (i.e., advantages of the hospitalist model)
- What the patient and family can do to maximize the chances of a good outcome from the hospital stay (e.g., follow-up with referring physician, compliance with prescribed treatments)

---

working relationship with the hospitalist. In other cases, it may be appropriate for the referring physicians to maintain some kind of involvement with the patient during the hospital stay. This may take the form of a single phone call to the patient or family, or one or more face-to-face visits, although this may be difficult given time constraints. No matter what the primary care physician's involvement is while the patient is hospitalized, distributing a hospitalist brochure to patients, either ahead of time during an office visit or at the beginning of hospitalization, is an important element of patient communication in hospitalist systems.

THE ROLE OF THE HEALTHCARE EXECUTIVE

The hospital's executive must have an understanding of the resources needed to allow optimal communication in hospital medicine programs (see Table 9.2).

ELEMENTS OF COMMUNICATION BETWEEN HOSPITAL LEADERSHIP AND THE HOSPITAL MEDICINE PROGRAM

As discussed in Chapter 14, the hospital medicine group's relationship with hospital leadership is a critical factor in determining the success of the program. In well-functioning hospital medicine programs, an effective relationship exists such that clinical and related administrative matters are addressed between the hospitalist medical director and the hospital leadership. For communication to be optimal, the following should take place:

- A representative from hospital leadership, usually the chief medical officer, should regularly attend hospital medicine group administrative meetings.

Table 9.2. Resources Needed for Effective Communication in Hospital Medicine Programs

Type of Communication	Resources
Between the hospitalist and the referring (or other involved) physician	• Rapid transcription of documents dictated by the hospitalists, including discharge summaries, histories and physicals, and consultations • Availability of a priority dictation line for hospitalists to perform stat dictations • Real-time faxing of dictated documents or electronic transmission of pertinent documents to referring physicians • A paper-based or electronic process for sending a complete list of discharge medications to the physician receiving a patient discharged from a hospital (Joint Commission requirement)
Between the hospitalist and the patient (and her family and significant others)	• Hospitalist brochure and marketing materials • Private areas on patient care units where discussions can occur
Among members of the hospital multidisciplinary team	• Conference rooms or office space near patient care areas • Allotted time
Among the hospitalists themselves	• Office space • Communication devices—pagers; cell phones; personal computer with laboratory, radiology, hospital information system, electronic billing, e-mail, and text messaging capabilities

• The hospitalist medical director should regularly attend hospital leadership meetings.

The key information that should be exchanged between the hospital leadership and the hospital medicine group is outlined in Table

Table 9.3. Communication Between Hospital Leadership and the Hospital Medicine Group

Information Flow	Type of Information
From hospital leadership to hospitalists	• Strategic goals of the hospital and/or employing entity • Regulatory and compliance issues • Patient safety and quality improvement initiatives • Operational issues that may affect hospitalists (e.g., information technology problems, lack of availability of specialists for emergency department call, changes in staffing in ancillary departments) • Financial goals and challenges for the hospital or sponsoring organization
From hospitalists to hospital leadership	• Barriers to collaboration with other departments (e.g., emergency department–hospital medicine group conflicts) • Hospitalist morale problems that may affect quality of care • Work environment issues that may adversely affect patient care (e.g., shortages of medical supplies, problems with clock synchronization or temperature control) • Work environment issues that may adversely affect the effectiveness of the hospitalists or other medical staff (e.g., lack of workspace, shortage of computers)

9.3. For a detailed discussion of elements of hospital medicine program performance that should be reported to hospital leadership, see Chapter 15.

CONCLUSION

A thoughtful approach to communication is an important determinant of hospitalist success in providing service to stakeholders. Healthcare executives and hospitalists share important responsibilities in understanding the scope of the communication challenge, supporting the establishment of a communication infrastructure, and allocating sufficient resources to address communication requirements.

REFERENCES

Dudas, V., T. Bookwalter, K. M. Kerr, and S. Z. Pantilat. 2001. "The Impact of Follow-Up Telephone Calls to Patients After Hospitalization." *American Journal of Medicine* 111 (9B): 26S–30S.

Isaac, D. R., A. J. Gijsbers, K. T. Wyman, R. F. Martyres, and B. A. Garrow. 1997. "The General Practitioner-Hospital Interface: Attitudes of General Practitioners to Tertiary Teaching Hospitals." *The Medical Journal of Australia* 166 (1): 9–12.

Joint Commission. 2007. *National Patient Safety Goals.* [Online information; retrieved 01/19/07.] www.jointcommission.org.

Lindenauer, P., S. Z. Pantilat, P. P. Katz, and R. M. Wachter. 1999. "Hospitalists and the Practice of Inpatient Medicine: Results of a Survey of the National Association of Inpatient Physicians." *Annals of Internal Medicine* 130: 343–49.

Nelson, J. R. 2001. "The Importance of Postdischarge Telephone Follow-Up for Hospitalists: A View from the Trenches." *American Journal of Medicine* 111 (9B): 43S–44S.

Pantilat, S. Z., P. K. Lindenauer, P. P. Katz, and R. M. Wachter. 2001. "Primary Care Physician Attitudes Regarding Communication with Hospitalists." *American Journal of Medicine* 111 (9B): 15S–20S.

ADDITIONAL READINGS

Goldman, L., S. Z. Pantilat, and W. F. Whitcomb. 2001. "Passing the Clinical Baton: 6 Principles to Guide the Hospitalist." *American Journal of Medicine* 111 (9B): 36S–39S.

Wachter, R. M., and S. Z. Pantilat. 2001. "The 'Continuity Visit' and the Hospitalist Model of Care." *American Journal of Medicine* 111 (9B): 40S–42S.

Whitcomb, W. F., R. Holman, and J. R. Nelson. In press. "Communication in Hospitalist Systems." In *Comprehensive Hospital Medicine*, edited by M. V. Williams. Philadelphia, PA: Saunders.

CHAPTER 10

Hospitalist Staffing

Key Message

Estimating the number of required hospitalists to staff a practice necessitates an analysis of projected workload and the work capacity of an individual hospitalist.

Many different methods can be used to develop an estimate or starting point for how many full-time equivalent (FTE) hospitalists are required to staff a particular practice. This chapter presents a reasonably quantitative three-step approach (see Figure 10.1). A review of several issues that could lead to modifying the original estimate will follow.

ESTIMATING FTE REQUIREMENTS FOR A PRACTICE

Step 1: Estimate Practice Workload

Workload for an existing practice should be assessed by obtaining or estimating annual totals for the following measures of patient volume:

Figure 10.1. Three-Step Process for Developing a Hospitalist Staffing Plan

1. Estimate practice workload (patient volume).
2. Analyze survey data on annual productivity output per hospitalist.
3. Divide the total anticipated work volume (Step 1) by the relevant annual productivity output per hospitalist (Step 2) to calculate the number of FTE hospitalists required.

FTE: full-time equivalent

- Number of new referrals, including admissions (inpatient and observation status) and consults (when the hospitalist is asked by other doctors to serve as a consultant)
- Procedures, such as lumbar puncture and central line insertion
- Work relative value units (wRVUs) generated
- Billable encounters

These metrics describe the direct patient care workload for a hospitalist and do not account for additional activities that many hospitalists provide, such as teaching, participating in a rapid response team, leading initiatives such as implementing computerized physician order entry, and participating in committee work. These other activities are addressed later in the chapter.

A new practice with no track record of patient volume can estimate patient volume by totaling the anticipated number of annual referrals in each of the following categories:

- *Referrals from primary care physicians (PCPs).* The hospital can survey PCPs regarding whether they plan to refer their patients when the hospitalist practice starts. For PCPs who plan to refer, historical admission counts can be obtained from the hospital's database. One caution: PCPs often underestimate the likelihood that they will refer, so the estimate from the survey may be lower than the reality.
- *Unassigned medical admissions from the emergency department.* Most hospitals can get historical counts of these admissions.

Hospitalists rarely serve as the admitting doctor for all unassigned admissions. For example, they are not usually expected to admit surgical or trauma patients. Hospitals vary significantly regarding which types of patients are admitted by hospitalists.

- *Perioperative consults.* Hospitalists are often asked by surgeons to provide preoperative assessments and perioperative care for medical issues. Most institutions do not have a way to reliably estimate this volume in advance, but anecdotal experience suggests it can range from 5 percent to 25 percent of the hospitalist workload.

- *Referrals from local specialists (i.e., doctors other than PCPs) and other hospitals.* Patient volume in this category can vary significantly from one practice to the next, ranging from none to as much as 30 percent of the overall hospitalist practice volume. This can be estimated by analyzing local referral and hospital transfer patterns.

Adding the estimated number of new referrals in each of the categories mentioned provides an estimated annual patient volume for a start-up hospitalist practice.

Step 2. Analyze Survey Data Regarding Productivity

Survey data should be reviewed with regard to typical patient volumes (outputs) per hospitalist. These may vary by practice type. Society of Hospital Medicine's (SHM 2006) biannual survey, *2005–2006 Compensation and Productivity Survey*, has the largest sample size and offers the most comprehensive information. Another source is the Medical Group Management Association's (MGMA 2006) *Physician Compensation and Production Survey.* Summary data from these two surveys are presented in Table 10.1.

In both surveys, productivity numbers vary significantly based on variables such as practice type (e.g., academic, community

Table 10.1. Key Survey Metrics of Hospitalist Productivity

Measure	SHM Survey*		MGMA Survey*	
	Mean	Median	Mean	Median
Annual new referrals	547**	468**	N/A	N/A
Annual encounters	2,458	2,328	1,913	2,025
Annual wRVUs	3,213	3,217	3,769	3,514

*Both surveys report data collected in 2005.
**Data from 2004 surveys (collected in 2003). The metric was not assessed in the SHM 2006 survey.
SHM: Society of Hospital Medicine; MGMA: Medical Group Management Association; wRVU: work relative value unit

based), geographic location, age of practice, and employment model (private group versus hospital employed). These numbers should not be regarded as the gold standard for a particular practice. Instead, they should serve as a starting point to determine the optimal workload per hospitalist. The right staffing may vary from one practice to the next, even if the practices have the same patient volumes.

Step 3. Calculate the Number of Hospitalists Required

To calculate the required number of hospitalists, divide the total anticipated work volume (step 1) by the relevant annual productivity output (step 2). The calculations to estimate the number of FTE hospitalists required for a practice are illustrated in Table 10.2. In this hypothetical case, these calculations, using three different metrics, show the practice needs between 4.8 and 5.7 FTEs.

These calculations provide a starting point for the analysis of hospitalist staffing. Several additional variables can be used to determine whether a practice needs more or less than the FTEs projected by this analysis.

Table 10.2. Calculating FTE Requirements for a Hypothetical Practice

Metric	Projected Annual Volume for Practice*	Output per Hospitalist from Survey**	FTEs Required (A ÷ B)
New referrals	2,750	547	5.0
Encounters	11,860	2,458	4.8
wRVUs	18,432	3,213	5.7

* Hypothetical numbers generated for illustration only.
** Numbers are means from the SHM 2006 survey.

OTHER APPROACHES TO ESTIMATING STAFFING REQUIREMENTS

Coverage Requirements or Hours Worked

Using the annual workload and hospitalist productivity calculations as described earlier is not the only way to project staffing requirements. Sometimes coverage requirements dictate the number of hospitalists required. For example, a practice may require 24/7 on-site coverage, with a hospitalist available around the clock. Even though the patient volume may indicate the need for only three hospitalists, the practice may require five hospitalists to provide the necessary coverage. For practices with eight or more hospitalists, the number of FTEs should be similar whether calculated based on workload or coverage. But for smaller practices, especially those staffed by less than three doctors, the two methods may yield significantly different results.

Daily Census

Most hospitalist literature and surveys report that a reasonable daily patient load is 12 to 18 patients. This is a worthwhile guideline, but staffing based on this metric alone can be problematic. For example, daily patient load can be defined as the census (the number of patients being treated) or as the number of daily billable encounters (which will yield a higher number than the census). Counting encounters is usually the better measure of workload.

However, staffing based solely on either daily billable encounters or patient census can be misleading because it reflects only one perspective of workload. As illustrated in Figure 10.2, a doctor who has high average daily encounters but works relatively few shifts yearly may have annual productivity below a doctor who has low average daily encounters but works more shifts in a year. It is important to recognize this trade-off between average daily encounters and number of annual shifts worked.

Rather than using patient census or daily encounters as the starting point for staffing decisions, it might be better to use it as a final

---

Figure 10.2. Which Hospitalist Has the Greater Workload?

Dr. A has an average daily census of 17
Dr. B has an average daily census of 13
• Using the metric of encounters per day, it appears that Dr. A has a greater
  workload.

But,
Dr. A works 7 on/7 off (183 days per year), resulting in 3,111 encounters
Dr. B works 240 days per year, resulting in 3,120 encounters
• Now, using the metric of encounters per year, it appears that Dr. B has a
  greater workload.

However,
Dr. A has an ALOS of 4.1 days, therefore seeing 759 admissions/discharges
Dr. B has an ALOS of 4.3 days, therefore seeing 726 admissions/discharges
• Using the metric of admissions per year, once again it appears that Dr. A
  has a greater workload

ALOS: average length of stay

---

test of whether staffing and scheduling decisions are reasonable. The preferred approach is to develop an estimate of required staff based on coverage needs and workload, then develop a work schedule, and finally assess the daily encounters that result from these calculations. While there is no recognized optimal number of daily encounters per hospitalist, anecdotal evidence suggests that most practices work best if a doctor rarely (e.g., no more than 10 percent of shifts) has more than 20 encounters in a day.

PRACTICE ATTRIBUTES THAT MIGHT INCREASE OR DECREASE FTE REQUIREMENTS

New or Very Small (≤3 Hospitalists) Practices

New practices often begin operations before they are fully staffed. In most cases, it is reasonable to start operating the practice (perhaps with a more limited scope of work at the outset) when the first hospitalist is available. The remaining staffing of hospitalists can often be made up by community doctors who are willing to moonlight on a temporary basis for the hospitalist practice. As each new hospitalist is hired, the need for moonlighters will decrease.

Some practices find that using part-time or moonlighting hospitalists on an ongoing basis can be useful. Particularly for small groups, part-time doctors or moonlighters make it easier to develop a sustainable work schedule for the full-time doctors.

Experience shows that start-up practices can often find PCPs in the area who are willing to moonlight. Many of these PCPs refer their patients to the hospitalists, but they will occasionally work for the hospitalist practice so that they do not lose their inpatient skills. Sometimes, about the same time the hospitalist practice has less need for moonlighters, the PCPs lose interest in moonlighting and prefer to work solely in the office setting.

It is reasonable to question whether part-timers or moonlighters in a hospitalist practice can provide care of the same quality and efficiency as the full-time doctors. To date, no formal research has been conducted on this issue, but anecdotal experience shows that many hospitalist practices incorporate part-time doctors successfully.

Rapid Volume Growth in New Practices

Patient volume in a brand-new hospitalist practice often grows very rapidly. In most cases, it is a mistake to assume that volume will "ramp up" slowly like it might for other physician practices. In fact, some practices can reach their projected mature patient volume within four to eight weeks of operation. There are examples of hospitalist groups in which the first hospitalists resigned because they were overwhelmed by the rapid growth in patient volume that outpaced the group's ability to add hospitalists. (See the discussion in Chapter 5).

Nonclinical Activities

As detailed in Table 10.3, hospitalists often have significant responsibilities in addition to direct patient care. Although the data do not include an estimate of the amount of time spent by hospitalists doing these nonclinical activities, it can be significant and may require additional hospitalists in the practice.

Scheduling Decisions

The issue of scheduling, as detailed in Chapter 11, is complex and can influence workload capacity, sometimes significantly. What might first be seen as insufficient hospitalist staffing (or excessive workload) may be a scheduling problem. Therefore, when addressing workload and staffing problems, it is important to consider ways that the hospitalists' schedule might be adjusted to better match

Table 10.3. Hospitalist Nonclinical Activities

Activity	Percentage of Hospitalist Groups Involved in the Activity
Committee participation	92
Quality improvement	86
Practice guideline development	72
Pharmaceutical/therapeutics committee	64
Utilization review	59
CPOE/information systems	54
Teaching—house staff	51
Teaching—non-MDs	36
Recruit/retain MDs	31
Community service	28
Disaster response/planning	25
Research	21

CPOE = computerized physician order entry
Source: SHM (2006).

staffing to workload. Adjusting the schedule might mean shortening or lengthening some work periods (shifts), adding new shifts such as an evening shift that handles only admissions and "cross cover" work, and varying the number of hours worked by each hospitalist from one day to the next to match each day's patient load.

Night Coverage for the Practice

While it may be counterintuitive, practices that have one or more daytime doctors available by pager at night have higher productivity per doctor than those that have a separate night shift. Consider a practice that has three doctors working each day and rotating responsibility for taking calls by pager from home at night. As the practice volume grows, nights on call go from being relatively quiet to nearly always requiring significant after-hours work and leading to sleep deprivation. The practice decides to switch from pager call at night to a dedicated night shift in-house. Making this change leads to an increase from three to four doctors working every 24 hours or the addition of .75 to 1.50 FTE hospitalists. But this increase in staffing occurs without an increase in patient volume (workload), so the average annual productivity per doctor goes down. Nonetheless, for many hospitalist practices, the benefits of a separate night shift may be worth the cost of some reduction in productivity per FTE. See Chapter 12 for a more extensive discussion of night coverage.

The Role of Allied Health Professionals

Nurse practitioners (NPs) and physician assistants (PAs) can be valuable members of the team in many hospitalist programs. As noted in Chapter 8, the SHM (2006) survey reported that 16 percent of hospitalist groups employ PAs and 20 percent employ NPs.

Hospitalist programs should consider going through a thoughtful process of analyzing whether or not they should add NPs or PAs. As part of this analysis, the group should carefully estimate the economic impact of adding an NP or a PA instead of a physician. Refer to Chapter 8 for specific strategies on how to deploy NP/PA staffing.

NONCLINICAL STAFF IN A HOSPITALIST PRACTICE

Administrative Support Staff

Most hospitalist practices should have clerical support to manage incoming phone calls from outside the institution and to assist with routine paperwork, including mail distribution and supporting the billing function. Smaller practices may require only half-time clerical support (e.g., a hospital employee who works full time and supports the hospitalist practice and another hospital department at the same time). Larger practices need full-time support.

Other Support Staff

Some practices include dedicated nurses who serve as rounding assistants to the doctors, dedicated case managers, and other clinical support staff. These roles are discussed in more detail in Chapter 8.

CONCLUSION

Each practice environment presents a unique situation with regard to the volume and nature of the patient workload and the definition of hospitalist responsibilities. A hospitalist medical director, often in conjunction with the hospital administrator, must develop an approach for staffing that is relevant to the specific hospitalist program.

REFERENCES

Medical Group Management Association (MGMA). 2006. *Physician Compensation and Production Survey.* Englewood, CO: Medical Group Management Association.

Society of Hospital Medicine (SHM). 2006. *2005–2006 SHM Survey: State of the Hospital Medicine Movement.* Philadelphia, PA: Society of Hospital Medicine.

CHAPTER 11

Hospitalist Scheduling

Key Message

The scheduling model used by a hospitalist group can have a significant impact on its performance and on physician satisfaction.

The previous chapter addresses staffing a hospitalist practice—that is, determining how many full-time equivalent providers a practice needs. This chapter discusses issues relevant to deciding how to schedule the providers to meet the practice workload demands while maintaining a healthy lifestyle for the doctors. Scheduling is a vital priority for a hospitalist program, affecting its economic health, clinical quality, and physicians' well-being.

Hospital executives should be aware that hospitalist scheduling is different from scheduling in most other forms of physician practice. Consider the following four issues:

1. *Unpredictable variations in work volume.* The volume of inpatient work can vary significantly and unpredictably from day to day, arguably more than in most other types of physician practice.

One day, the work volume might be 70 percent of the average, and the next day it could be 140 percent of the average. There is no way to reliably predict these variations when creating a work schedule.

2. *Around-the-clock responsibilities.* Significant patient care demands arise 24 hours a day, 7 days a week. There is usually just as much work on weekends as on weekdays. A significant portion of the daily work must be done after hours (e.g., between 6 p.m. and 7 a.m. the next day).

3. *Importance of continuity.* Hospitalist–patient continuity over the course of the patient's in-hospital stay is important. Patient care suffers when too many handoffs occur. This must be taken into account when creating the hospitalist work schedule. Although emergency physicians must deal with unpredictable demand and around-the-clock responsibilities, the issue of continuity adds another layer of complexity to the challenge of scheduling hospitalists.

4. *Interplay between schedule and staffing needs.* The choice of schedule has a significant influence on productivity and staffing needs. A situation that appears to be a staffing problem may really be a problem of poor scheduling (e.g., patient volume might dictate the need for six hospitalists, but because of poor scheduling choices, the practice appears to need seven hospitalists).

Hospitalist groups vary substantially in their scheduling issues. It might be said that no two groups have the same scheduling requirements. However, each hospitalist group should evaluate its schedule, using the checklist provided in Figure 11.1, to ensure that it is effectively supporting the group's goals.

ELEMENTS OF HOSPITALIST SCHEDULING

Six key elements or decision points should be considered when developing a schedule for a hospitalist practice:

Figure 11.1. Checklist for Evaluating a Hospitalist Schedule

Patient Care
- Does the schedule risk compromising the quality or safety of patient care?
- Does the schedule provide for reasonable patient–hospitalist continuity?
- Does the schedule provide for a reasonable patient load per doctor?*

Physician Lifestyle
- Does the schedule allow sufficient time off?
- Does the schedule provide for flexibility of time off (i.e., time off when desired rather than just when schedule provides it)?
- Are worked days/nights routinely too short or too long?
- Does the schedule require a doctor to change from day work to night work too often?
- Does the schedule provide for an equitable number of weekends worked?
- How does the group perceive the burnout risk of the schedule?
- Does the schedule have a way to handle sudden absences (e.g., illness)?

Flexibility
- Does the schedule allow for adjusting staffing in response to varying patient loads?
- Does the schedule anticipate how additional doctors will be added to the schedule?

Business Operations
- Does the schedule optimize production capacity of available hospitalists?
- Does the schedule account for nonclinical activity, such as committee work?

* In measuring patient load per doctor, use daily encounters rather than the average daily census. Also, look at more than the averages. Think about how often a doctor's patient load exceeds what is regarded as the maximum "safe" daily load.

1. Number of consecutive days worked
2. Length of each worked day (or night)
3. Number of worked days (and/or nights) annually
4. Bimodal distribution of workload over each calendar day
5. Night work
6. Weekend work

Number of Consecutive Days Worked

Handoffs of patients from one hospitalist to another should be minimized; ideally, a patient should see the same hospitalist each day. Good continuity between patient and hospitalist is likely to lead to many benefits, including improvements in patient satisfaction and fewer errors arising from "fumbled" handoffs. A hospitalist is typically not very efficient when taking over responsibility for the patients of a colleague who is to be off for the next few days. A handoff requires taking the time to get to know each of the patients. Working more consecutive days minimizes the frequency of such handoffs, and the hospitalist can safely see more patients in less time.

Of course there is a limit to the number of consecutive days a hospitalist can work. Each group needs to determine the trade-off between maximizing continuity and burning out physicians by having them regularly work an unreasonable number of days in a row. Many practices schedule doctors to work between 5 and 14 consecutive days, separated by nearly as many days off. Some practices provide excellent continuity by routinely having hospitalists work as many as 21 consecutive days, but this requires a schedule in which some of the worked days will be very short.

Length of Each Worked Day (or Night)

A tension exists between the length of each worked day and the number of consecutive days the doctor can work; lengthening one will usually require shortening the other. Many hospitalist groups work a schedule based on fixed shifts. The shift length is often set at 12 hours, because that might be the longest period that a doctor could work day after day without burnout. It also creates a schedule in which day shifts and night shifts are of equal length. While this is a frequently used model and a reasonable approach, other models may be better. Some groups choose to schedule shorter day shifts (e.g., 10 hours) and longer night shifts (e.g., 14 hours), especially if the nights are not routinely busy and might offer a chance to rest or sleep. If nights are routinely busy (e.g., in a large practice), then it would be reasonable to shorten the night shift and have one or more day-shift doctors work more than 12 hours or to add an evening shift (described in more detail below).

A schedule based on shifts of a predetermined fixed duration is common for hospitalists. It provides a predictable lifestyle for the doctor and a known amount of hospitalist hours for each day. But because practice workload varies considerably from one day to the next, this rigidity can lead to frequent mismatches between workload and staffing. One way to more closely match each day's hospitalist staffing level to workload is to minimize fixed-duration shifts so that the hospitalists adjust the number of hours they work each day according to the demand. See Figure 11.2 for the benefits and drawbacks of eliminating fixed start and stop times for shifts.

Number of Worked Days (and/or Nights) Annually

An important variable in developing a hospitalist schedule is how many days or shifts each doctor will have to work annually. Society of Hospital Medicine's 2006 survey data (collected in 2005) show that hospitalists using a schedule of fixed-duration shifts worked a median of 188 11-hour shifts annually, and those who had on-call responsibilities in addition to regularly scheduled shifts worked a median of 215 days annually.

Figure 11.2. Pros and Cons of Eliminating Fixed Start and Stop Times for Day Shifts

Pros
- Daily hospitalist staffing levels can be adjusted to match workload.
- Some working days can be made shorter than a fixed-duration shift schedule, thereby
  - making it possible to work more consecutive days to maximize continuity;
  - potentially preventing burnout, because not every worked day is long (as is the case in a 12-hour fixed-shift schedule); and
  - making it easier to work more days annually (which may increase productivity and participation in other hospital activities, such as committees).
- Hospitalists can take more control over the pace of their work (e.g., when they start and stop, how long can they take for breaks).

Cons
- The hospitalist may be out of the building in the afternoon when the patient deteriorates and needs to be seen again. (Note that this drawback can be partially addressed by requiring all hospitalists to stay on pager until the night shift starts and by requiring that at least one doctor stays in the hospital at all times.)
- The impact on personal lifestyle is less predictable (e.g., it is hard to know exactly when a physician will be home each day).
- A month's schedule is more complicated to create than if all shifts are identical.

There is no right number of days or shifts a hospitalist should work annually. However, it is important to acknowledge that to achieve an annual productivity target (e.g., the SHM [2006] survey median for work relative value units), a hospitalist who works fewer days in a year will need to do more work each day (e.g., maintain a higher census or number of daily encounters) to achieve the same productivity as a hospitalist who works more days in a year.

Bimodal Distribution of Workload Over Each Calendar Day

A factor often not considered when developing a schedule is that, for most practices, the workload peaks in the morning from roughly 7 a.m. to noon, when rounding is done, and again between 3 p.m. and 11 p.m., when most new referrals/admissions (usually from the emergency department) need to be seen. Schedules often address the workload peak for rounding but face a problem from about 6 p.m. to 11 p.m., when workload, primarily in the form of new admissions, may require more than the one scheduled on-call or night hospitalist.

To illustrate this problem, think of a practice that has four hospitalists who arrive to work each morning at 7 a.m., work 12 hours, and then all sign out, leaving a single night doctor working a 12-hour night shift, starting at 7 p.m. In all likelihood, on many days there will be more admissions for the first few hours of the night shift than the night hospitalist can safely handle, resulting in a frustrated or burned-out doctor and delays in seeing emergency patients.

One way to address this problem is to have one of the day hospitalists stay on duty until 8 p.m. or 9 p.m. every fourth day so that there will be at least two hospitalists available during that time (i.e., the day hospitalist who stays late and the night hospitalist). This is an efficient use of hospitalists and other clinical staff, but it can be unreasonably taxing for a doctor to work such a long day in a busy practice. Another approach is to add a new evening shift into the scheduling model. This could be scheduled from late afternoon to sometime near midnight, thereby extending two-hospitalist coverage until later in the night. However, this model requires the financial cost of adding another hospitalist in each day's schedule and adversely affects continuity because patients admitted by the evening doctor will nearly always be handed over to another doctor the next morning.

Night Work

While significant variation exists, it is reasonable to estimate that 10 percent to 20 percent of the work in a hospitalist practice occurs between 6 p.m. and 7 a.m. the next day. For small practices (e.g., fewer than six full-time doctors), it can be reasonable for hospitalists to work a series of consecutive days while rotating night call taken by pager from home and returning to the hospital at night as needed. However, this means there will not be a hospitalist in the building 24 hours a day. Dedicated in-hospital night coverage for such a small practice is expensive, but some hospitals may believe the investment is warranted.

Once a practice has grown to roughly six or more hospitalists or is admitting two to three patients per night, dedicated night coverage is advisable. In scheduling dedicated night coverage, the night hospitalist should have no responsibility to the practice during daytime hours on the day before or after. (Working consecutive nights while off during the daytime is reasonable.) It is important to realize that this transition from a traditional "beeper call from home" system of night coverage to providing dedicated in-hospital coverage will likely lead to a paradoxical decrease in productivity per hospitalist (and therefore a *decrease* in the profitability of the overall program and additional support dollars from the hospital or other sponsoring organization). While the night work makes major demands on the hospitalist (e.g., sleep deprivation and burnout), it will not generate as much professional-fee revenue as daytime work. Experience indicates that night work generates professional-fee revenue as efficiently as day work when seven to eight new referrals/admissions come in during every night shift (typically, for a hospitalist practice of 15 to 20 physicians).

Although it is expensive to support a system in which a doctor has no responsibility to the practice the day before or the day after a night shift, it also carries many benefits. Specifically, it is likely to lead to improvements in burnout, career satisfaction, and longevity for hospitalists. While not proven, it probably also leads to improved quality and efficiency of care by providing an alert hospitalist who expects to be working, rather than relying on a doctor awakened at night to practice medicine via the telephone. Furthermore, a night hospitalist may lead to improved job satisfaction for night nurses. Chapter 12 provides a more detailed discussion of night coverage arrangements.

Weekend Work

For most hospitalist practices, weekends are just as busy as weekdays, making it difficult to reduce weekend staffing. Most practices choose to staff weekends with the same number of providers as weekdays. Furthermore, implementing a schedule that treats weekends (and holidays) like other work days is good for hospitalist–patient continuity. But in many cases, such a system may mean that a full-time hospitalist has to work about half the weekends of a year.

Some strategies can be used to reduce the number of weekends an individual hospitalist is on duty, but they are problematic. One approach is to use part-time doctors (e.g., office-based doctors who moonlight for the hospitalist practice) or dedicated "weekendists" who work only on weekends to replace full-time doctors on some of the weekends. Another approach is to simply reduce staffing on weekends, recognizing that hospitalists will accept being busier on weekends in exchange for working fewer of them. Unfortunately, both of these strategies have an adverse impact on continuity, and using moonlighters or weekendists is usually expensive. Still, some practices choose to use one or both of these strategies, believing that their cost is worth the perceived benefit in physician well-being and recruiting.

PUTTING IT ALL TOGETHER

Mapping a Doctor's Schedule

After considering the six elements described earlier and other requirements that may be unique to a particular hospitalist practice, the work schedule for each hospitalist needs to be mapped out on a calendar. Many groups use a model of x consecutive days of work followed by Y days off in a fixed, repeating pattern. This has the advantage of making it easy for a doctor to forecast well in advance which days will be spent working and which will be days off. However, an often unrecognized downside to this approach, especially when each worked day is a fixed-duration shift (e.g., always 12 hours), is that a hospitalist may increasingly tend to segregate his professional life from his personal life. During their sequential days of work, hospitalists may minimize social activities such as going to dinner with friends or activities like exercise or chores at home. They may try to limit all such personal activities only to their days off. This "systole-diastole" lifestyle may over time lead to increased resentment of work and burnout.

An alternative approach is to vary the number of consecutive worked days and the number of consecutive days off. This may discourage segregation of one's work and personal life in such a systole-diastole fashion. It also has the benefit of allowing each doctor to try and schedule time off when he wants it, rather than in a rigidly repeating manner. Sometimes the doctor may be happy to have only two or three days off and then return to work, and at other times she may want two weeks off. This kind of flexibility is difficult to achieve with a schedule based on fixed, repeating intervals.

Hospitalists in university teaching hospitals often approach scheduling differently. There are many situations in which they are responsible for patient care one month at a time, and on other months they are engaged in research and other academic activities. In this case, they may work nearly all of the days of their month "on service" (including weekends), and any vacation or extra time off is scheduled for the other months.

7-On/7-Off Schedules

The most common hospitalist scheduling format is probably a schedule of seven consecutive worked days, followed by seven off.

In most cases, each worked day is scheduled as a 12-hour shift. There are a number of reasons for the popularity of this model:

- It is easy to understand and mark out on the calendar.
- Having 26 weeks off every year is very attractive for recruiting.
- It provides for reasonably good hospitalist–patient continuity of care.

The popularity of this approach suggests that it is a reasonable choice for many groups. However, each group should consider the costs of this kind of schedule and ensure they do not exceed its benefits. These costs include the following:

- A potentially unhealthy systole-diastole segregation of professional and personal life may result, as discussed earlier. This may increase burnout.
- The schedule results in working relatively few days annually. Working 7 out of every 14 days means 182.5 worked days annually (or less if there are additional vacation days) and requires much higher patient volumes per worked day to yield typical hospitalist productivity. For comparison, doctors in a practice who each works 220 days annually could have the same annual productivity with 17 percent fewer average daily visits.
- Having every other week off gets in the way of each hospitalist being involved in hospital activities that do not follow a similar alternate week schedule, such as committee work.

CONCLUSION

There is significant variation in what constitutes a reasonable work schedule for hospitalists. Hospitalists in the practice should have input in developing their schedule. However, hospitalist group leaders and hospital executives involved with the practice should have a fundamental understanding of the important scheduling issues discussed in this chapter. A poorly designed schedule can lead to physician dissatisfaction and burnout, as well as inferior clinical and economic outcomes. A well-designed schedule should prevent these problems and should be flexible and adaptable to changing work demand and practice volume. Even if a practice has what is regarded as an optimal schedule now, it is likely that it will require significant modifications as the practice grows.

REFERENCE

Society of Hospital Medicine (SHM). 2006. *2005–2006 SHM Survey: State of the Hospital Medicine Movement.* Philadelphia, PA: Society of Hospital Medicine.

ADDITIONAL READINGS

Mistry, B., and W. Whitcomb. In press. "Scheduling and Staff Deployment for Hospital Medicine Programs." In *Comprehensive Hospital Medicine*, edited by M. V. Williams. Philadelphia, PA: Saunders.

Nelson, J., and W. Whitcomb. 2002. "Organizing a Hospitalist Program: An Overview of Fundamental Concepts." *Medical Clinics of North America* 86 (4): 887–909.

CHAPTER 12

Night Coverage for Hospitalist Practices

Key Message

Night coverage in a hospitalist practice is expensive and difficult to staff. It requires careful planning, implementation, and budgeting.

A common reason that hospitalist practices struggle or fail is the design of their night coverage. Both executives and practicing hospitalists should think carefully about their approach to night work. This chapter highlights several important issues to consider.

Society of Hospital Medicine (SHM 2006) survey data (collected in 2005) show that 51 percent of hospitalist practices have a provider in the hospital at night. Compared to groups providing on-call night coverage from home, these practices are more likely to be hospital employed and working in a hospital with more than 100 beds. Figure 12.1 reveals a trend away from call-based (on call from home) and toward shift-based scheduling.

Table 12.1 shows additional SHM 2006 survey data regarding night coverage arrangements, specifying the types of hospitalists that are on-site overnight.

Figure 12.1. Scheduling Paradigms

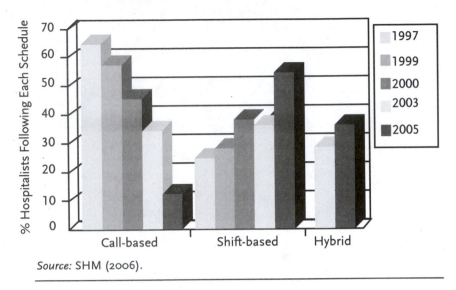

Source: SHM (2006).

Table 12.1. Night Coverage Arrangements for Hospitalist Programs

Type of Night Coverage	Percentage of Hospital Medicine Groups
On-site providers	51
On-call hospitalists from home	41
No night coverage	8
For the 51% of groups* that have an on-site provider, that provider is a:	
Physician hospitalist	95
Contracted physician (e.g., moonlighter)	24
Physician nonhospitalist (e.g., resident/fellow)	11
Physician assistant	5
Nurse practitioner	3

*Groups can use more than one type of provider
Source: SHM (2006).

A framework describing the structure of night work for a hospitalist practice is described in Table 12.2. It features four attributes or decision points:

1. Is a hospitalist in the hospital all night?
2. Does the hospitalist working the night shift typically work the previous or subsequent day shift?
3. Does the compensation amount or methodology differ for day work and night work?
4. Do hospitalists who work nights also work days?

In general, nearly any combination of these variables is possible, and each group will need to decide the best approach individually.

COMMON ARRANGEMENTS FOR NIGHT WORK

Small practices, such as those with fewer than five to six full-time hospitalists, and practices that are in a start-up phase usually provide night coverage via a traditional on-call arrangement. In this coverage arrangement, one of the day doctors remains on call at night to do work as required and returns to work the next day. The volume of night work in small practices is often too low to justify a dedicated night-shift arrangement.

A common approach for a larger practice is to have a system of dedicated night shifts in which the night hospitalist does not work the day before or after working a night. Typically, the night shifts are divided equally among all providers in the practice, unless some members of the group prefer nights.

Some practices are able to staff most or all nights with nocturnists—hospitalists who only work nights. To employ nocturnists, usually night compensation, shift length/frequency, or patient load is set appealingly enough that some providers are attracted to night work. The benefit of this approach is that the day doctors will not need to rotate back and forth from day to night work.

Table 12.2. A Decision Framework for Night Coverage Arrangements

Decision Attribute		Comments
Is a hospitalist in the hospital all night?	Yes	Very expensive for smaller practices, but has many benefits; usually essential for large practices
	No	Usually means call from home by pager (traditional on call) or one night doctor covering more than one hospital
Does the hospitalist working the night shift typically work the previous or subsequent day shift?	Yes	Usually means call from home by pager in a small practice only (traditional on call)
	No	Best described as dedicated night shift to distinguish from traditional on-call system (i.e., work today, on call from home tonight, work tomorrow)
Does the compensation amount or methodology differ for day work and night work?	Yes	Allows providers in practice to be flexible and not insist that each work the same portion of nights (It can be worthwhile to set night compensation [or shift length/ frequency or patient load] appealingly enough that providers are just as attracted to night work as day work.)
	No	Usually realistic only when each provider works an equal portion of nights
Do hospitalists who work nights also work days?	Yes	A common arrangement (An individual doctor might work two to seven consecutive nights, then have some days off and return to the day schedule for a few weeks before repeating the cycle.)
	No	Doctors who only work nights (nocturnists) can provide a number of benefits for a practice

Roles for night hospitalists most commonly include the following:

- Admitting patients referred to the hospitalist practice
- Providing hospitalist consultative services as requested by other doctors
- Handling nursing calls regarding issues related to patients who are the responsibility of day hospitalists (i.e., cross coverage)
- Caring for emergent or urgent patient care issues, such as rapid responses, code blues, or other unstable patients

NIGHT HOSPITALIST COMPENSATION

If all hospitalists provide an equal amount of night coverage in rotation (e.g., each member of a four-person group works 61 nights annually), then adjusting the compensation scheme to reflect night work is not necessary. Providing a night-shift differential in this situation will not influence an individual doctor's annual income relative to his partner hospitalists.

However, if the hospitalist program seeks to create more flexibility, it may be advisable to provide more income for a night of work than a day of work. Under this scheme, hospitalists may voluntarily trade day and night work among themselves, leading to enhanced satisfaction (e.g., Dr. A is willing to work some of Dr. B's nights because of the income benefit. Dr. B may or may not work some of Dr. A's days in return).

If the practice has one or more dedicated nocturnists, then the nocturnists will need to realize some benefit to working only nights. This benefit can take many forms, such as the following:

- The night hospitalist works less often than the day doctors (e.g., day doctors work 220 days annually, while night doctors work 182).

- The night hospitalist has a lighter patient load (e.g., a night hospitalist in a small practice typically sleeps three to six hours per night shift, while the day doctors typically work a busy 8- to 12-hour shift).
- The night doctor has a higher income than the day doctors.
- The night doctor has a higher priority in time-off scheduling.

It is common to combine these benefits. For example, a night hospitalist might work less often than the day doctors, have a lighter patient load, and have the same annual income. Anecdotal experience shows that a higher income or working less often than day doctors is valued more than a reduction in patient load.

For most practices, compensating hospitalists based significantly or entirely on their production can be a good idea, but it might be problematic for a night doctor. It could lead the night doctor to encourage marginal admissions to the practice, some of whom will need to be discharged by the daytime hospitalists hours later. In effect, the night hospitalist could say, "I'll admit anyone I can get my hands on since my income will increase. I'll leave it for the day doctors to sort out what to do with all these patients." In addition to being poor patient care practice, this would be inefficient for the hospital and the hospitalist practice.

PRACTICE ECONOMICS RELATED TO NIGHT COVERAGE

A traditional system of night call (such as pager call from home while also working days) is usually less expensive than a system of dedicated night shifts. Consider the following example:

- On any given day, a hospitalist practice with five full-time equivalents (FTEs) has three doctors working, one of whom will be on call that night by pager.

- That will mean 219 worked days per year for each doctor (3/5 × 365), one-third of which (73) will be spent on call. Each hospitalist gets 146 days off per year.
- The practice decides to switch to a system of dedicated night shifts in which the doctors do not work during the day before or after a night shift. The practice wants to retain the 146 days off for each hospitalist. This new coverage arrangement is equivalent to adding 365 new shifts annually (one for each night).
- This will require an additional 1.67 additional FTE hospitalists (1.67 hospitalists at 219 shifts/year = 365).

In the example described, by switching from on-call coverage to on-site coverage, the practice increased from 5 FTEs to 6.67 FTEs. If the daytime work was already enough to keep all three doctors busy, then adding 1.67 FTEs to allow dedicated night shifts may not significantly increase the practice productivity or revenue. In that case, the practice looks much less productive per FTE (6.67 FTEs are now seeing the same volume that was previously handled by 5 FTEs) and much more costly.

It is worth emphasizing this point: *Changing from a system of traditional night call to dedicated night coverage does not usually increase the practice workload capacity significantly.* Instead, it offers other benefits, such as those listed in Figure 12.2. Some practices find that they must provide for dedicated night coverage to recruit hospitalists effectively. Other institutions choose to support it, believing it leads to more timely and efficient care that is also of higher quality.

Despite the high cost of a system of dedicated night coverage or nocturnists, most practices should plan to incorporate it into their practice at some point. As an individual practice's patient volume grows, it is increasingly unreasonable for the hospitalists to handle nights via a traditional on-call system. On-call coverage results in poor sleep for the doctors, which may result in increased errors and decreased career longevity.

Figure 12.2. Potential Benefits of Dedicated Night Coverage

- Enhanced career satisfaction and longevity for hospitalists (less burnout)
- Improved hospitalist recruiting
- Potential to implement other night initiatives, such as hospitalists serving on code response or rapid response teams
- Improved quality of care through eliminating the need for patients to be admitted by the emergency physician (or by the hospitalist by phone without being seen) with long delays until the patient is seen in person by the hospitalist
- Modest improvement in revenue possible by billing admissions before midnight rather than the next day
- Improved night nurse satisfaction, because they have access to an awake doctor who is expected to be working rather than having to page and wake up a doctor who is trying to sleep

Once a practice requires six to seven daytime providers working each day, or has 16–20 new admissions/referrals daily, then the volume of work on a night shift may be enough that a single night doctor might be as productive (e.g., as measured in work relative value units) as a day doctor. This can make the night shift as cost effective as the day shift. However, some nights will be much busier than average, and the night doctor may be overwhelmed such that some of the benefits listed in Figure 12.2 are lost.

HOW TO INCREASE THE PRODUCTIVITY OF NIGHT WORK

Smaller practices that want to implement a system of dedicated night shifts or nocturnists but are concerned about low night-shift patient volumes and professional-fee revenue might want to explore ways to make the night shift busier and more financially productive. One option is to consider having the night hospitalist take on additional responsibilities on behalf of other (nonhospitalist) physicians. In some cases this could mean the following billable activities:

- Admit patients for all members of the medical staff (as long as this can be done safely given the nocturnist's residency training). For example:
  o A primary care physician (PCP) typically cares for all his hospitalized patients and does not refer to the hospitalists. One of his patients needs admission at night. The nocturnist could do a full history and physical, write an admission order (not just a holding order), and turn the patient over to the PCP the next morning.
  o At 2:00 a.m., the emergency department (ED) refers to a surgeon a patient with abdominal pain who might need a cholecystectomy. The surgeon tells the ED doctor by phone, "I'll accept the patient on my service. Have the nocturnist admit the patient to me." The nocturnist does a full history and physical and writes an admission order on behalf of the surgeon. Note: A patient suspected of having a problem requiring urgent specialty evaluation would not be referred to the nocturnist (e.g., for a patient who may or may not require urgent surgery, the surgeon's input is needed to make that decision).
- Provide internal medicine/primary care consultative services as requested by other doctors. For example:
  o An orthopedist did a knee replacement on a relatively healthy patient of a PCP who does not refer to hospitalists. Hospitalists have not been involved in the care of the patient, and the patient's PCP has not seen the patient during this admission (i.e., has not been consulted by the orthopedist). During the night the nurses report to the orthopedist that the patient has suddenly become short of breath. The nocturnist sees the patient, does a complete consultation, and provides the care the patient needs. The

next morning the nocturnist lets the patient's PCP know what has happened, at which point the PCP takes over. Note that the day hospitalists are not involved with this patient at all.

- Handle nursing calls regarding medical issues arising on all patients in the hospital. For example:
  o The nurse calls the nocturnist first for patients with the following types of issues: a surgeon's patient needs a sleeping pill, an oncologist's patient has very elevated blood pressure, a patient on the rehabilitation unit has a fever, a gastrointestinal doctor's patient has become hypotensive, and so forth. If the patient issue proves to be complicated, the nocturnist calls in the attending physician to see the patient.

The expanded responsibilities just described may not be attractive for a nocturnist. However, it might enable an attractive salary for the nocturnist while working far fewer shifts annually than might be required for daytime work. It is also a way for a hospital to fully use the night hospitalist, provide benefits for all of the medical staff, and mitigate the increasing stress of on-call work for many specialties.

If the nocturnist submits charges for all billable visits, she generates some of the revenue required to support her position. This means that those community doctors who have the nocturnist admit or consult on patients at night may lose the chance to bill for those services themselves. Thus, each doctor who has the nocturnist treat her patients gives up some professional-fee revenue to support the program.

CONCLUSION

Night work is one of the most stressful parts of a hospitalist's career and one of the most challenging problems for leaders of a hospitalist practice. There are many potential benefits of a system of dedicated night shifts, but for small practices such a system is likely to be seen as prohibitively expensive. However, over the long run, dedicated night coverage is likely to be an important component of a successful hospitalist practice. Each practice will need to think carefully about how to make its system of night coverage cost effective.

REFERENCE

Society of Hospital Medicine (SHM). 2006. *2005–2006 SHM Survey: State of the Hospital Medicine Movement*. Philadelphia, PA: Society of Hospital Medicine.

ADDITIONAL READINGS

Mistry, B., and W. Whitcomb. In press. "Scheduling and Staff Deployment for Hospital Medicine Programs." In *Comprehensive Hospital Medicine*, edited by M. V. Williams. Philadelphia, PA: Saunders.

Nelson, J., and W. Whitcomb. 2002. "Organizing a Hospitalist Program: An Overview of Fundamental Concepts." *Medical Clinics of North America* 86 (4): 887–909.

CHAPTER 13

Hospitalist Compensation

Key Message

The most effective compensation scheme for hospitalists should include meaningful incentives for production and quality.

The *amount* of hospitalist compensation—how much a hospitalist should make—and the *method* by which hospitalists are paid—specifically, a fixed salary or compensation that includes incentives—are key decision points in developing a hospitalist practice. In addition, three special issues are related to compensation: (1) paying for night coverage, (2) compensating hospitalist medical directors, and (3) transitioning to new compensation schemes.

Hospitalist compensation has been rising over time. The explosive growth of the specialty has undoubtedly contributed to this trend. Because the demand for hospitalists exceeds the available supply, employers are often willing to offer higher compensation to recruit hospitalists. In the late 1990s the most common method of hospitalist compensation was a straight (fixed) salary, but in the last few years a move has been seen toward other methods that connect a portion of the compensation to production and/or performance on quality metrics.

SOURCES OF REVENUE FOR HOSPITALIST PRACTICES

Funding for most hospitalist practices comes from two sources: professional-fee revenue and some other source—usually the hospital. Society of Hospital Medicine (SHM 2006) survey data (collected in 2005) show that 97 percent of hospitalist practices reported receiving financial support in addition to professional-fee collections. The amount of this additional support averages 25 percent of the practice budget, or an average of $550,000, which works out to approximately $60,000 per full-time hospitalist annually. Figure 13.1 shows typical figures for a prototype hospitalist based on the 2005 SHM data.

Figure 13.1. Financial Averages for a Typical Hospitalist

Revenue

Professional-fee collections	$200,000
Additional revenue (typically from the hospital)	$60,000
Gross Revenue	**$260,000**
Overhead (estimated at 18.8% of total revenue)	($48,880)
Net Revenue	**$211,120**
Expenses	
Hospitalist salary	$169,000
Benefits	$27,656

Source: SHM (2006).

AMOUNT OF HOSPITALIST COMPENSATION

The two most useful surveys of hospitalist compensation are the biannual SHM survey and the annual survey published by the Medical Group Management Association (MGMA 2006). While both are valuable sources of data, it is worth understanding some important ways in which they differ:

- The data in the MGMA survey tend to come from large physician organizations and probably underrepresent hospital-employed programs and smaller, local, private hospitalist groups. Close inspection of the MGMA data shows that many hospitalists report a large volume of outpatient visits, suggesting that there may be significant commingling with data from doctors in traditional (hospital and office) practice.
- The SHM data capture a larger number of hospitalists and, unlike the MGMA data, are the result of a survey designed specifically for hospitalists. However, because the aggregate data come from all types of hospitalist practice (e.g., academic and community hospital hospitalists, as well as those who work for corporate, multistate companies), it is worth taking the time to drill down into the SHM data to find results that most closely match a particular work environment.

Table 13.1 compares data from the SHM and MGMA surveys.

Several other organizations publish survey data on hospitalist compensation, but these surveys usually focus on a narrow market segment, such as one part of the country. *Modern Healthcare* magazine aggregates data from many of these surveys in an annual physician compensation issue published each July (e.g., Romano 2006).

Figure 13.2 shows the historical trend in hospitalist compensation, using SHM survey data. Some of the upward trend in income is probably explained by factors such as inflation, but the survey

Table 13.1. SHM and MGMA Productivity and Compensation Data*

	SHM Data		MGMA Data	
	Average	Median	Average	Median
Compensation	$169,000	$168,000	$189,403	$182,184
Benefits	27,656			
Annual productivity				
Encounters	2,548	2,328	1,913	2,025
Work RVUs	3,217	3,213	3,769	3,514

*Data for both surveys were collected in 2005 and reported in 2006.
Note: The MGMA survey reports a significant number of outpatient visits attributed to hospitalists, but the number of encounters shown in this table is for inpatient visits only. The work relative value unit numbers in the MGMA data apply to both inpatient and outpatient encounters. The SHM survey combines all encounters that hospitalists report, while the MGMA data do not. These issues probably account for much of the discrepancy between the two survey results. See Table 4.2 for medians of hospitalist compensation by region, experience, specialty, and employment model.

shows rising levels of productivity for individual hospitalists, as measured in annual encounters or relative value units (RVUs), which probably accounts for some of the increase in compensation. It is important to note that changes in the survey population from one year to the next might confound the data. For example, many more academic hospitalists, who tend to have lower annual incomes, appear in the later surveys than the earlier ones.

In January 2007 the Centers for Medicare & Medicaid Services (CMS) adopted a revised RVU scale, which increases the RVUs assigned to many of the Current Procedural Terminology (CPT) codes used by hospitalists. For many practices, the revised scale will result in an increase of approximately 10 percent or more in professional-fee collections. As this book goes to press, it remains to

Figure 13.2. Median Hospitalist Compensation, 1997–2005

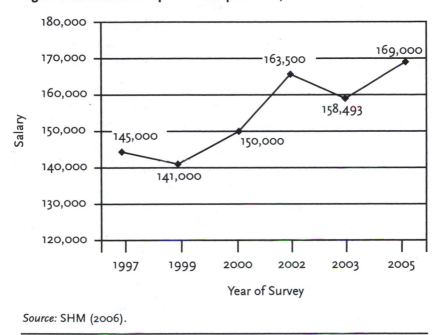

Source: SHM (2006).

be seen whether this will lead to a commensurate increase in hospitalist incomes.

It is important to emphasize that there is significant variation in all of the compensation and productivity metrics and that survey data, whatever the source, should not serve as the sole guide regarding appropriate compensation for a particular practice. A more meaningful benchmark may be the compensation of doctors in the local marketplace with the same training who are in traditional practice. Anecdotal evidence indicates that hospitalists who care for adult patients (usually trained as internists) make roughly 5 to 15 percent more than internists in traditional practice (office and hospital) in the same market. Factors that can lead to hospitalist salaries that are significantly higher than survey results include higher-than-average productivity and/or a significant shortage of hospitalist staffing in a region.

METHOD OF HOSPITALIST COMPENSATION

There is no one best method to compensate hospitalists, but a practice should seek to implement a plan that meets the following criteria:

- *Is easy to understand.* It should be easy for the doctors and administrators connected to the practice to describe how the compensation system works and the rationale behind it.
- *Is easy to defend in public.* A good compensation plan should not cause embarrassment or concern if other hospital personnel, patients, or a malpractice jury learn how the compensation system works.
- *Complies with all laws and regulations.* It must be within fair market value and meet other standards. This may require review by legal personnel.
- *Can be modified over time.* A practice should anticipate that, over time, the schedule and the way work is distributed among providers may change significantly. It is best if a compensation plan does not need to be rewritten every time such changes are made. Ask the following question: Will the plan still work well if the practice adds more providers and implements a schedule that is significantly different from the current schedule?
- *Rewards good work.* Ideally, the compensation methodology should support the practice goals and encourage the doctors to think of themselves as owners of the practice, even if they are contractors. Any variable or incentive component of compensation should be large enough to influence behavior, and incentive targets should be set so that they are not too easy or unreasonably difficult to achieve.

Since the mid-1990s, the straight, or fixed, annual salary approach to compensation has given way to an approach that combines fixed and variable components. The common methods of hospitalist compensation can be grouped into three broad categories, as reflected in Table 13.2 and discussed in the next section.

Straight or Fixed Salary

Compensating hospitalists using a fixed salary method was popular in the 1990s because it was simple to understand and budget. Also, it can significantly facilitate recruiting, because doctors who have just completed residency are attracted to the notion of a guaranteed income. However, a straight salary approach offers no reward for good performance and is inflexible, such that changes in the number of providers or in workloads have no impact on compensation. This can encourage the doctors to disconnect decisions about how hard they work and how much money they make. They may see the best day of work as one in which they have no new referrals. They may be unreasonably quick to want to add providers in response to modest or temporary increases in patient volume. Under the straight salary approach, hospitalists may not understand the economic realities of the practice. Their employer likely will have an economic incentive to have them work longer hours and see more patients. This can lead to the doctors and the employer having different points of view about the costs and benefits (financial and otherwise) of staffing and workload decisions.

Table 13.2. Portion of Hospitalist Groups Using Each Compensation Method

Compensation Method	Percentage of Practices Using Each Method
Fixed + variable salary components	68
Straight salary (no variable component)	27
Based entirely on production	4

Source: SHM (2006).

Additionally, under a fixed salary, the doctors have no personal economic incentive to ensure that they are capturing all charges and choosing CPT codes optimally. In many practices, this leads to poor charge capture (some visits go unbilled) and/or undercoding that results in lower professional-fee revenue for the practice. And other doctors (nonhospitalists at the institution) may view the hospitalists as less service oriented if they know that the hospitalists' work decisions (e.g., which patients they do and do not accept) have no influence on their income.

Despite its simplicity and benefit for recruiting, a straight or fixed salary usually proves problematic and undesirable for most hospitalist practices. Most practices should avoid this method in favor of some variable compensation system (discussed later) but may want to offer an income guarantee (or floor) for the first one or two years a doctor is in the practice. This guarantee should usually be set below what that doctor's income is projected to be from the standard (variable) salary method.

Combining Fixed and Variable Salary Components

According to the SHM 2006 survey data, most hospitalist practices compensate the doctors based on some combination of a base (or fixed) salary component and a variable component based on some metric such as production or quality metrics.

For most groups, the purpose of the variable salary component is to motivate and reward good performance, thereby addressing some of the shortcomings of the fixed salary. Its effectiveness is a function of two attributes:

1. *The portion of overall compensation connected to the variable component.* Some practices connect only a small amount (e.g., less than 5 percent) of total compensation to the variable component. This may be too small to significantly motivate physician behavior. A doctor is unlikely to focus on performance on a

particular quality metric if her compensation is affected by only $2,500 annually. Instead, she is likely to practice as usual and hope that things work out well enough to get all of the $2,500 at the end of the year. But if $25,000 of compensation is at risk, it is likely to significantly influence the doctor's behavior.

Similarly, the amount of the variable compensation can affect the willingness of a hospitalist to work harder. If the practice connects only a small portion of compensation to productivity, then each extra unit of work (e.g., each additional patient, wRVU, or encounter) pays incrementally less. So while the hardworking doctor would earn more than others in the practice, the incremental increase in salary would be unreasonably small. The hardworking doctor's average compensation per unit of work would be lower than that of the doctors who do not work as hard.

2. *Whether the variable component is connected to metrics that are too easy or to hard to achieve.* If the work required to earn all of the available variable compensation is perceived as impossibly hard or exceptionally easy, the doctor will probably not pay much attention to it. A group might decide to reward good performance on CMS core measures (e.g., giving pneumovax to patients with pneumonia), but if the physician is required to have a 100 percent compliance rate to earn the variable compensation, then he is likely to ignore it.

A more common error is to set the target unreasonably low. If the doctor's historical rate of appropriate pneumovax administration is 60 percent, it will be of little value to implement a variable salary component that offers a financial reward for a rate of 65 percent. It is often best to adopt a sliding scale approach in which each percentage point of improvement results in a corresponding percentage of the total variable compensation available to the doctor. In other words, the portion of the total available variable component dollars is a function of the degree of improvement seen. This avoids having to negotiate an all-or-none threshold for payment.

Table 13.3 characterizes the metrics used in incentive compensation, based on the SHM 2006 survey of hospitalist programs. Production incentives (e.g., wRVUs) can be a good way to ensure that each doctor is personally connected to the economic health of the practice. Quality incentives help ensure attentiveness to optimal practice patterns and clinical decision making. It may be best to use a compensation model that includes quality- and production-based incentives. For example, a doctor might earn an annual fixed base salary of $70,000 and have a variable component based on production projected to result in $70,000 (e.g., $21.88 paid for each wRVU generated in a practice where the average doctor generates 3,200 wRVUs annually) and up to $50,000 for optimal performance on a few quality indicators.

Note that a variable component based on production is best connected to each doctor's individual performance. But for many

Table 13.3. Metrics Used in Incentive Compensation for Hospitalists

Metric	Percentage of Hospitalist Practices
Production metrics (e.g., RVUs, charges, encounters, admissions)	82
Quality metrics (e.g., CMS core measures, patient satisfaction)	61
Committee or project work	16
Teaching	3
Medical records completion	1
Longevity (years worked)	1
Other	6

Note: 290 of 396 surveyed practices (73 percent) reported using an incentive compensation approach. The percentages in the table reflect the proportion of the 290 groups using the specified incentive metric. Data collected in 2005.

Source: SHM (2006).

quality metrics, it can be difficult to attribute performance to an individual doctor (e.g., who gets the credit or blame for a patient's pneumovax if three hospitalists cared for that patient?), and the metrics are best based on the group's performance as a whole such that each doctor gets the same share of the incentive payment. If a quality metric is easy to attribute to a particular hospitalist, then an individual incentive makes sense. Whatever metric is chosen, it should be relatively easy to measure. Some groups have tried to implement compensation components tied to a variable, such as the time of day a discharge order is written. That is a worthwhile idea but can prove labor intensive to measure, and it may be very difficult to resolve any disputes about the accuracy of the data. The best metrics are those that are already being measured and for which the hospitalists have confidence in the accuracy of the data.

When choosing quality metrics it is important not to dilute the dollars available by too many metrics. For example, it may be reasonable to decide to make up to $15,000 available annually for good performance on quality metrics, but it could be counterproductive to tie it to 20 separate metrics such that excellent performance on each would pay less than $1,000. In general, it is best to limit the number of metrics and align them with those for which the hospital is being held accountable to the best extent possible.

Compensation Based Entirely on Physician Productivity

Only 4 percent of hospitalist practices report having compensation based entirely on production (SHM 2006), despite the fact that it is probably the most common method of compensation for physicians (regardless of specialty) in the United States. The low percentage is probably a result of several concerns, including that it creates incentives to do more rather than to do better. However, because physician productivity is a critical component of the economic health of every hospitalist practice, it remains a reasonable method for compensating hospitalists.

The drawbacks to compensation based entirely on production include the following:

- It is difficult to implement in a new hospitalist practice because no track record has been established of what patient volumes will be. This problem can be mitigated by offering a doctor an income guarantee or floor for the first year or two.
- It offers a financial reward to a hospitalist who decides to work an unreasonable amount, potentially paying less attention to quality.
- Compensating based on metrics that are influenced by length of stay (e.g., wRVUs, encounters, charges, collections) can misalign the hospital and physician economic incentives by paying the doctors more for keeping patients in the hospital longer.
  o Note: This problem can be avoided by using a case-rate compensation, which pays a fixed amount to the doctor for each new referral (admission or consult) accepted into the practice regardless of how many subsequent visits the doctor makes.
- Hospitalists themselves are often reluctant to connect a significant portion of their income to production because they have limited control over how hard they work from one day to the next. However, workload can be predicted reasonably well over any long period (e.g., a year) by the doctors' decisions on staffing and scheduling.
- Hospitalists may be concerned that they will have to compete with one another for patients, thereby disrupting the collegial relationship that is so important to any group. However, experience shows that this is an uncommon problem, and in the rare case it occurs it usually reflects excessive staffing (or insufficient patient volume) rather than an indictment of productivity-based incentives.

While no good survey or research data are available to show how prevalent these problems are, anecdotal experience suggests that they are usually not significant enough to make productivity-based compensation unreasonable for hospitalists. It has a number of significant benefits, including the following:

- It is usually relatively simple to administer.
- It liberates the doctors in an individual practice to work different amounts and, within some boundaries defined by the group, to make individual choices about what is the "sweet spot" between workload and income.
- It will encourage the doctors to be more flexible in their scheduling decisions. Rather than thinking of their compensation as being connected only to the number of shifts or hours they work, hospitalists will have an economic reason to continually fine-tune their work schedule to provide for optimal distribution of hospitalist resources.
- It encourages the doctors to take into account all variables related to their staffing decisions. Because they will be assuming some personal financial risk, administrators will know why hospitalists have included financial issues in their staffing decisions.
- It encourages the doctors to think of themselves as owners of the practice, even if they are in fact employees of an organization like a hospital or a large group practice. Productivity-based compensation can help prevent the doctors from having an attitude of "I've been hired to work just this many shifts at this salary, and it is someone else's problem to work out the finances."

When paid on production, hospitalists gain some freedom to adjust how much they work; it may mean a doctor can choose to work less than was required under the fixed-salary method. Of course the group as a whole will still need to get all of the work done, but they will have more flexibility to trade work among the hospitalists or decide to increase (or decrease) their overall staffing to achieve what they regard as the optimal combination of workload and income.

Table 13.4 illustrates some concepts that can be useful when designing the structure of an incentive compensation scheme that includes both production and quality components. The table suggests some schemes that can be implemented under three different compensation models—productivity based, productivity and quality incentives, fixed salary with quality incentive.

Table 13.4. Sample Approaches to Incentive Compensation

	Fixed Component (Base Salary)	Production Incentive (Assume 3,200 wRVUs/Year/Doctor)	Quality Incentive
100% productivity-based compensation	0	$53.12 per wRVU (= $169,984)	
Productivity and quality incentives	$100,000	$21.85 per wRVU (= $69,920)	Up to $20,000 per doctor based on five quality metrics (max. $4,000 per metric); sometimes best structured so that each member of the group is paid same portion of the incentive based on the group's overall performance
Fixed base salary with quality incentive	$150,000	$0	$20,000 per doctor structured as described above

SPECIAL SITUATIONS

Compensation for Night Shifts

Night work may require a different compensation amount and method than day work. For example, the day work could be paid at $X per wRVU and the night work could be paid at $1.5X per wRVU, or the night work might include a higher base rate in addition to the productivity compensation. See Chapter 12 for a more detailed discussion of compensation for night shifts.

Compensation for Group Leaders

SHM (2006) survey data show that hospitalist group leaders earned an average of $11,000 more annually than nonleader hospitalists, although the amount varies significantly from practice to practice. A good approach is to combine an increase in compensation and a reduction in clinical time to provide time for administrative activities. A rough rule of thumb is to reduce the group leader's clinical time by 5 percent of a full-time equivalent (FTE) for each FTE in the practice. Thus, in a ten-physician group, the leader might work 50 percent of a clinical FTE, and in a 15-physician group, clinical time might be reduced to 25 percent. Of course the compensation of a group leader should reflect the perceived talent and value of that particular person. See Chapter 14 for details on the role of the hospital medicine group director.

Transitioning to a New Compensation Scheme

Hospitalist groups should periodically examine their compensation system and evaluate the pros and cons of alternative approaches. When a group decides to change the compensation system, it usually takes a number of meetings (among the hospitalists and with the hospitalists' employer) spread over several months to reach an agreement. It is helpful to run reports that show what each doctor would have earned if the proposed new system had been in place.

During the first year of any new compensation system with a variable component, it is advisable to provide each doctor with a reasonable guaranteed income. For example, if a new system is based on productivity, and the average doctor in the group is expected to earn $175,000 annually, the practice might offer a one-year income guarantee set at around $165,000. That approach will address much of the perceived risk of the new system as well as will preserve the doctor's incentive to perform well.

CONCLUSION

There is no one-size-fits-all approach to compensating hospitalists. A common error made by hospitals and hospitalist programs is to link the compensation plan too tightly to the group's staffing and scheduling system. This will result in either (1) the need to adjust and rewrite the compensation formula or (2) resistance to making adjustments in the staffing and scheduling approach (such as number and length of shifts) as the need arises.

Most groups should consider connecting a significant portion of compensation to productivity. It is not unreasonable, and can be worthwhile, for nearly 100 percent of compensation to be tied to production, although for most hospitalist programs the productivity component is in the 10 to 20 percent range. Also, the compensation approach in many practices should include incentives tied to quality metrics (which might change as often as every year). To be effective, quality incentives should be substantial, representing 5 percent or more of total compensation.

The targeted total annual compensation for hospitalists should consider survey data, but more importantly it should reflect the structure of the practice and the local marketplace. Many factors could justify compensation higher or lower than the survey data; the most important one is differences in workload between a particular practice and the survey data.

REFERENCES

Medical Group Management Association (MGMA). 2006. *Physician Compensation and Production Survey.* Englewood, CO: Medical Group Management Association.

Romano, M. 2006. "Bigger Payday for Some Docs." *Modern Healthcare* (July 17): 26–30, 34.

Society of Hospital Medicine (SHM). 2006. *2005–2006 SHM Survey: State of the Hospital Medicine Movement.* Philadelphia, PA: Society of Hospital Medicine.

ADDITIONAL READINGS

Holman, R., W. Whitcomb, and J. Nelson. In press. "Compensation Principles and Practices." In *Comprehensive Hospital Medicine,* edited by M. V. Williams. Philadelphia, PA: Saunders.

Nelson, J. 2006. "SHM 2005-06 Compensation and Productivity Survey Results." Presentation at the Society of Hospital Medicine Annual Meeting, Washington, DC, May 4–5.

CHAPTER 14

The Role of the Hospital
Medicine Group Director

Key Message

The hospitalist medical director is perhaps the single most important determinant in the success or failure of a hospital medicine program.

The medical director is the linchpin of the hospitalist program and the most important individual member of the hospital medicine group. In programs that enjoy a great deal of success, a strong group leader is invariably at the helm. In programs that are struggling, the most common thread is the lack of strong leadership. Indeed, few operational or strategic challenges cannot be overcome with an effective medical director. On the other hand, even the most sound operational plan is prone to failure if no one is available to provide leadership in its implementation. A sample job description for a hospitalist medical director is presented in Appendix F.

MANAGING RELATIONSHIPS

Because hospitalists have a major impact on the acute care hospital and constantly interact with myriad stakeholders, the director's central task is to manage relationships. Such management requires the ability to balance a number of priorities simultaneously and to continuously direct and facilitate interactions with patients, families, and members of the hospital clinical and administrative teams. Figure 14.1 lists the most important relationships for the medical director. Ideally, the director should also relate to other key parties, such as the hospital's medical executive committee and the hospital's board of directors.

HIRING A HOSPITAL MEDICINE GROUP DIRECTOR

The director is the most important hire for the hospital medicine group. Because of the relative shortage of qualified leaders, it is vital to offer a competitive compensation package, especially when recruiting for the position. In terms of total compensation, the Society of Hospital Medicine (SHM 2006) productivity and compensation survey reports that hospitalist medical directors earn an average of $11,000 more than their nonleader hospitalist counterparts. To

---

Figure 14.1. Key Relationships for the Hospital Medicine Group Director

- Patients, families, and their loved ones
- Referring physicians
- Other members of the medical staff, including medical subspecialists and surgeons
- Hospital executive team, especially the chief medical officer
- Hospital clinical team—nursing, case management, therapy departments, etc.
- The hospital medicine group itself
- The public

---

get an effective hospitalist leader may require a higher level of investment. Local and broader market conditions dictate the total compensation required to recruit and retain a qualified leader.

When recruiting for a hospitalist director, look for someone who has the following background:

- A strong reputation in the local community
- Prior hospitalist experience
- A record of professional development in physician leadership

The ideal hospitalist group director is a physician who combines a broad vision with strong interpersonal, managerial, and clinical skills. Figure 14.2 lists key attributes of a hospital medicine group director.

KEY RESPONSIBILITIES OF THE MEDICAL DIRECTOR

The director has a broad array of responsibilities, both clinical and nonclinical. Figure 14.3 lists these responsibilities, and they are discussed in greater detail in the following section.

Figure 14.2. Important Attributes of the Hospital Medicine Group Director

- Strong interpersonal skills, including the ability to communicate, see others' points of view, and compromise while maintaining principles
- Good depth of character, including integrity, consistency, discipline, and follow-through
- Strong clinical skills
- Ability to work alongside, and advocate for, rank-and-file physicians
- Willingness to delegate important tasks
- Experience as a negotiator
- Ability to transform criticism into opportunities
- Understanding of the strategic direction of the employing entity (e.g., hospital, medical group)

Figure 14.3. Responsibilities for the Hospital Medicine Group Director

Clinical
- Provides direct patient care
- Leads quality and system improvement within the group and across the hospital
- Defines the scope of service of the hospital medicine group
- Oversees all group clinical decisions with the goal of minimizing substandard care
- Reviews individual hospitalist performance
- Reviews group performance with regard to quality of care, satisfaction, and efficiency metrics
- Handles complaints regarding the group

Nonclinical
- Works with and supervises the practice manager
- Provides the link between hospital administration and the hospital medicine group
- Educates medical staff and hospital staff about the role and limits of the hospitalists in clinical care
- Implements the strategic and competitive plans of the hospital, as appropriate
- Develops the strategic plan for the hospital medicine group, including marketing, growth/recruiting, service, and quality
- Oversees all financial aspects of the hospital medicine group, including budget development, revenue maximization, coding documentation, and expense management
- Develops and implements operational processes, including scheduling, staffing, communication, and census/workload management

CLINICAL RESPONSIBILITIES

While the medical director has a broad range of nonclinical responsibilities, the most important attribute for an effective hospital medicine leader is excellence in clinical practice. First and foremost, exemplary clinical practice gains credibility for the hospital medicine leader in the eyes of the medical staff. Conversely, a leader will be severely limited if her clinical skills are less than superb. An effective hospitalist leader should function clinically as a hospitalist for a substantial portion of his total time, such that hospitalists are subjected to the same work conditions as the rank-and-file physicians. It is in this capacity that an understanding of the nuances of hospital medicine practice is continually maintained.

In addition to direct patient care responsibilities, hospitalist leaders also have high-level clinical oversight responsibilities related to the hospital medicine program. These responsibility areas are documented in Table 14.1.

NONCLINICAL RESPONSIBILITIES

The nonclinical responsibilities of the medical director fit into three main categories: strategic, financial, and operational.

Table 14.1. Main Areas of Clinical Oversight for the Medical Director

Role	Responsibility
Quality assurance officer for all hospital medicine group patients	With the goal of eliminating substandard care, oversees all clinical decisions made by members of the hospital medicine group and provides appropriate feedback and corrective action to individual hospitalists
Definer of scope of clinical services provided by the hospital medicine group	Works with hospital administration, the medical staff, and the hospital medicine group to define and set boundaries for clinical services offered by the hospital medicine group to balance stakeholder requirements
Quality improvement officer for all hospital medicine group patients	Defines and implements, with key collaborators, best clinical practices through care standardization approaches such as guidelines, protocols, prompts, incentives, education, and alerts
Reviewer of clinical performance of each member of hospital medicine group	Periodically reviews the clinical practice profile of each hospitalist, based as much as possible on measurable, objective indicators of quality of care

Strategic

A major portion of the medical director's role is strategic in nature. He must construct a cohesive strategy that balances the competitive marketplace needs of the hospital with the requirements and perspectives of the hospitalists and the hospital medicine group. The needs of the broader medical staff must also be considered. Of course, any effective strategy places the welfare of the patient as paramount.

To understand the strategic direction of the hospital, the director must establish a strong connection with the executive leadership team. The director should regularly attend key hospital leadership team meetings and maintain current knowledge of the hospital's important initiatives. One of the critical links between the hospital medicine group and hospital administration lies in the relationship between the chief medical officer and the hospitalist medical director. A structured approach to this relationship is key, and a portion of the regular meetings between the two should be devoted to the hospital medicine group's role in carrying out the strategic priorities of the hospital. Finally, as a central element of the medical staff, the group director should ideally have a presence on the hospital's medical executive committee.

Financial

The hospitalist medical director is responsible for managing the hospital medicine group's budget. The budget is the vehicle for deploying staff and other resources in such a way that optimizes the performance of the group. The director is accountable to the hospital executive team—the chief financial officer, the chief operating officer, and/or the chief medical officer—regarding budget adherence and performance.

In the course of financial oversight of the group, the director will regularly review group and individual professional fee billing and charge capture. She should have regular contact with the group's biller to assess the billing process, from the submission of a bill to the time of collection. Beyond billing, the director should be aware of the status of all other revenue sources, including capitated payments, stipends, and other monies. It should be made clear that the director conducts financial oversight with the support of the hospital medicine group's practice administrator. The administrator carries out much of the detailed analysis so that the director can then conduct higher-level oversight.

Operational

The hospitalist leader is responsible for operational processes, including communication, scheduling, staffing, recruitment, census/workload management, and all other aspects of operations. While responsibility for operations can and should be delegated to other hospitalists and the practice administrator, the director must have up-to-date working knowledge of the status of all practice operations.

POSITIONING THE MEDICAL DIRECTOR FOR SUCCESS

Even the strongest medical director will not be fully effective if he does not receive the necessary support and resources from the hospital leadership to carry out essential duties. The following three elements of support must be in place to achieve success:

1. Sufficient administrative time
2. A practice manager and clerical help
3. Political support—within the hospital medicine group, the medical staff, and the executive team

Furthermore, larger hospital medicine groups should consider creating the position of an assistant medical director.

Administrative Time

What is the appropriate allocation of administrative time for the hospitalist director? This is a frequently asked question. It depends on a number of factors, including the maturity of the program, the level of infrastructure support, the size of the program, and whether other group members are assisting with administrative functions (such as scheduling, overseeing quality improvement for the group, or recruiting). A general guideline for calculating administrative time is as follows:

> 0.05 full-time equivalent (FTE) administrative time per 1.0 FTE hospitalist (e.g., a group with 10 FTE hospitalists needs 0.5 FTE administrative time for the leader)

This guideline may be adjusted up if the practice requires substantial time to develop operational policies and infrastructure, and it may be adjusted down if the practice is mature, runs smoothly, and does not require much time investment in infrastructure.

Administrative Support

Larger hospitalist groups benefit from having a practice manager who partners with the medical director in overseeing the nonclinical functions of the group. The role is akin to that of any medical group practice manager. The practice manager leverages the time and effort of the director by doing the following:

- Arranging and attending important meetings, recording minutes, and providing timely follow-up
- Working as a liaison with key stakeholders, including patients/families, hospital administration, the group itself, and the medical staff

- Helping to develop and disseminate group operating policies
- Assisting the director with personal schedule management

Political Support

The hospital executive team and hospitalist medical director will be most effective when they take steps to ensure that the director does not stand alone in the charged political environment that is often found in hospitals and hospital medicine groups. A number of reasonable approaches can be taken to support the medical director in this capacity.

- *A hospitalist oversight or steering committee* can be created, composed of members of hospital administration and the medical staff, to ensure good service, high-quality hospitalist care, and even-handed referral relationships with the medical staff. If executed well, this body can leverage the work of the medical director in balancing the needs of hospital administration and the medical staff with those of the hospital medicine group itself. It is especially effective in young programs where uncertainty surrounds issues related to quality, service, and referral patterns.
- *A hospitalist leadership council* can be established, composed of members of the hospital medicine group who can advise the medical director in political and administrative matters. To the extent that the director can only be successful if she has the trust and support of the group, this council serves to deflect some of the political responsibility away from the director and diffuse it among members of the group. If managed well, it may achieve greater group buy-in and cohesiveness.
- *A hospitalist compensation committee* can be constituted, consisting of members of the hospital medicine group. It provides the hospitalists with a formal mechanism to have input regarding how and how much they are paid. The committee's

purpose is to achieve broad hospital medicine group support regarding compensation, and it can be an extension of the hospitalist leadership council.

CONCLUSION

The hospital medicine group director arguably carries the greatest responsibility for the success of the hospital medicine group, and as such needs to be positioned for success to the greatest extent possible. Providing appropriate support for the group director is a core function of the hospital executive team, and the elements of such support are discussed here. This chapter focuses on the management functions of the group leader; however, it is in the artful execution of these functions that true leaders are born and developed.

REFERENCE

Society of Hospital Medicine (SHM). 2006. *2005–2006 SHM Survey: State of the Hospital Medicine Movement.* Philadelphia, PA: Society of Hospital Medicine.

ADDITIONAL READINGS

Dichter, J. R., and L. E. Cowan (eds.). 2003. *The Hospitalist Program Management Guide.* Marblehead, MA: HCPro, Inc.

Dressler, D. D., M. J. Pistoria, T. L. Budnitz, S. C. McKean, and A. N. Amin. 2006. "The Core Competencies in Hospital Medicine." *Journal of Hospital Medicine* 1 (suppl. 1): 76–77.

Holman, R. In press. "Leadership in Hospital Medicine." In *Comprehensive Hospital Medicine*, edited by M. V. Williams. Philadelphia, PA: Saunders.

Nelson, J. R., and W. F. Whitcomb. 2002. "Organizing a Hospitalist Program: An Overview of Fundamental Concepts." *Medical Clinics of North America* 86 (4): 887–909.

CHAPTER 15

Measuring Hospitalist Performance[1]

Key Message

Hospital leaders should work with their hospitalist medical director to develop a comprehensive performance reporting system or "dashboard" that includes utilization, productivity, clinical, and satisfaction measures.

The following ten metrics, identified by the Society of Hospital Medicine (SHM 2006), represent a starting point for hospitalist practices that wish to develop a comprehensive performance monitoring and reporting process. Each hospital medicine group can then choose what to measure, based on the priorities of the practice and its hospital or other sponsoring entities.

1. Volume data
2. Case mix
3. Patient satisfaction
4. Length of stay
5. Hospital cost and ancillary utilization
6. Productivity measures
7. Provider satisfaction

Figure 15.1. Ten Key Performance Metrics for Hospitalists

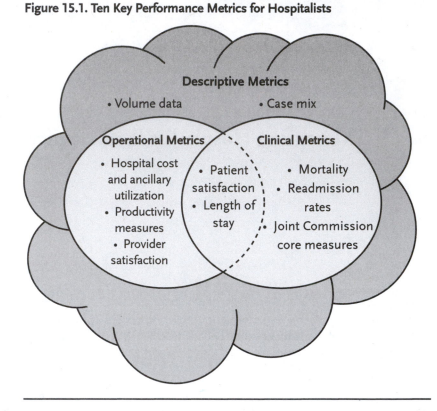

8. Mortality
9. Readmission rates
10. Joint Commission core measures

As illustrated in Figure 15.1, these metrics can be characterized in one of three categories: descriptive, operational, and clinical.

Volume and case mix are considered descriptive metrics because they do not measure hospitalist performance in and of themselves, but they inform, support, and explain the analysis of operational and clinical metrics. Operational metrics include items such as hospital cost, productivity (by individual physician and by group), and provider (usually referring physician) satisfaction. Clinical metrics include mortality, readmission rate, Joint Commission core measure compliance,

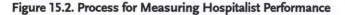

Figure 15.2. Process for Measuring Hospitalist Performance

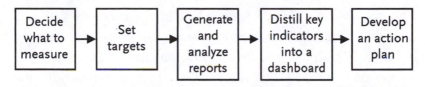

and similar items. Metrics such as patient satisfaction and length of stay may be considered measures of both operational and clinical performance.

To achieve effective performance monitoring, each practice should undertake a process similar to that outlined in Figure 15.2. Each step is discussed in the following section.

Decide What to Measure

In deciding what metrics to measure, consider the following questions:

- What were the original drivers for developing the hospital medicine group?
- What does the hospital (or other sponsoring organization) expect to achieve in return for its financial support?
- What do patients, payers, regulators, and other stakeholders want to know about the program?
- What are the high-priority issues currently confronting the practice?

Set Targets

Once a practice has decided on its basic metrics, it must set performance targets or goals so that the practice can measure its actual performance against desired targets. Such targets may be expressed as a floor (or ceiling) threshold, such as "at least 85 percent pneumovax compliance," or an ideal range of performance, such as "case mix–adjusted average length of stay between 3.2 and 4.0 days."

Generate and Analyze Reports

The practice must know where to obtain the necessary data and understand enough about how the data are collected and reported to be confident in the degree of accuracy and validity. Often, the required information is generated from hospital information systems, and the reports are voluminous and full of extraneous data items that make it difficult to focus on the key findings. It is important that the practice take the time to work with the individuals generating the data to create the most useful reports possible, to review and analyze the reports in detail on a regular basis, and to fully understand what the reports are saying about the practice and its performance.

Distill Key Indicators into a Dashboard

Because reports are often complex, voluminous, and overly detailed, it is important to select a handful of key business indicators, perhaps 10 to 20, and to summarize them in a dashboard.

A dashboard is a summary document, usually one to two pages long, that displays the most important practice performance indicators. It should be produced on a regular basis, such as monthly or quarterly, and it should display the key indicators in a simple, easy-to-read format that allows readers to quickly discern whether or not actual performance for the reporting period met the targets. The dashboard may include the following:

- The target performance level or range as well as the actual performance for each indicator, and/or
- A graphic display of
  o the performance trend over time, perhaps indicated by up and down arrows
  o whether actual performance meets the target for each indicator—for example red, green, and yellow lights

When deciding what to include in a dashboard, consider the following questions:

- What single parameter or item of information is the best indicator of the practice's performance for the metric under consideration?
- Which key parameters need to be monitored on a regular or ongoing basis, as opposed to on an as-needed basis, to know whether the practice is meeting its goals?
- Which parameters are essential for guiding the practice in taking actions to improve its performance in core areas?

Sample dashboards for a hospitalist program are presented in Appendix G.

Develop an Action Plan

The primary reason for measuring performance is to identify opportunities to improve it. Both detailed performance reports and the summary dashboard create opportunities to adopt a mind-set of continuous performance improvement. Secondary reasons for measuring performance may include demonstrating the value created by hospital medicine programs as follows:

- Documenting different levels of performance by hospitalists compared to a nonhospitalist peer group
- Calculating a return on investment for the hospital or other sponsoring organization in terms of improved quality and resource utilization or incremental patient volume and revenue

In summary, it is important to have a specific action plan for how the performance-monitoring information and the summary dashboard will be used to make decisions, improve performance, and demonstrate value. Questions to be addressed in developing the action plan should include the following:

- With whom will this information be shared? In what format will it be presented?
- What specific steps should be taken to improve performance for individual metrics?
- How will decisions be made about performance improvement priorities and resource allocation?
- How will this information be used to help further the interests of the hospital medicine practice?

CONCLUSION

A hospitalist program is accountable to many stakeholders, including hospital administrators, other physicians, patients, and the hospitalists themselves. A successful hospitalist program will implement a formal approach to performance reporting so that the group has a sense of accountability. This chapter has provided concrete suggestions on how to address the challenge of measuring hospitalist performance and use the information to attain better outcomes.

NOTE

1. The material in this chapter is excerpted from an unpublished white paper entitled "Measuring Hospitalist Performance: Metrics, Reports, and Dashboards," prepared in August 2006 by the Society of Hospital Medicine's Benchmarks Committee and Leslie Flores, coordinating writer.

REFERENCE

Society of Hospital Medicine (SHM). 2006. *2005–2006 SHM Survey: State of the Hospital Medicine Movement*. Philadelphia, PA: Society of Hospital Medicine.

CHAPTER 16

Hospitalist Information Systems

Key Message

Hospital leaders will need to invest in information system infrastructure to support a successful hospitalist program.

Like all organizations, hospital medicine groups need information systems to support daily operations and performance reporting (see Figure 16.1). However, hospital medicine groups by definition operate within the larger organizational structure of the hospital. Thus, hospitalist operational processes and reporting mechanisms, the information system infrastructure, must integrate with and take advantage of the hospital's information systems. The medical director of a high-performing hospital medicine group will be well versed in a hospital's clinical, financial, and analytical computer applications.

The following discussion examines hospitalist information systems from two perspectives:

1. *Basic:* the simple data-collection systems that should be implemented in start-up hospital medicine groups

Figure 16.1. Hospitalist Processes Supported by Information Systems

Operational Processes

- Scheduling
- Charge capture
- Clinical management
- Communications

Performance Reporting

- Service volumes
- Budgeting/financial reporting
- Utilization analysis
- Quality metrics
- Satisfaction surveys

2. *Sophisticated:* innovative information systems that have been developed and implemented by "advanced" hospital medicine groups and technology vendors

BASIC HOSPITALIST INFORMATION SYSTEMS

All start-up hospital medicine groups should implement simple data-collection systems. By way of example, this section outlines four manual processes and/or reports that a start-up group should consider implementing:

- Hospitalist log book
- Daily census report
- Charge capture system
- Primary care physician (PCP) communication system

Hospitalist Log Book

A sample hospitalist log book is shown in Figure 16.2. The log book is best maintained electronically (e.g., using an Excel spreadsheet). Each line in the log represents a hospitalist "case" (e.g., admission, observation, consultation, code blue) that includes the following data elements (Goldsholl 2006):

Figure 16.2. Hospitalist Log Book

Hospital Medicine Program

Date _____

Office Notified	H&P Sent	Admit Date	Patient #	Admitting MD	Referring MD	Diagnosis	D/C Date	Follow Up	D/C Sent

H&P: history and physical; D/C: discharge

- Patient identifier (medical record number)
- Type of case
- Admission date
- Referring physician (if available)
- Admitting physician/hospitalist
- Diagnosis
- Confirmation that office was notified
- Confirmation that history and physical (H&P) was sent
- Discharge (D/C) date
- Confirmation that discharge summary was sent
- Patient follow-up requirements

The electronic hospitalist log book can be used to support several processes for a hospital medicine group. First, it can provide a reference on the services performed by the hospitalist and allows reconciliation against the hospital's information system. This is important, as the hospital's information system will be a source of performance reporting (e.g., length of stay), and it is vital that hospitalist cases are accurately identified for analytical purposes. Second, it can provide accurate information on the referral source for hospitalist cases. Third, it can provide a common reference database for the hospitalists on cases they are treating or have treated. Finally, the hospitalist log book can provide a control mechanism to ensure that necessary information (i.e., the H&P and the discharge summary) is communicated to the primary care physician.

Daily Census Report

A sample daily census report is shown in Figure 16.3. Each line represents a day of the week, indicating the group's total workload for the day.

The first two columns of the daily census report indicate the starting census for the day—how many patients were being cared

Figure 16.3. Daily Hospitalist Census Report

Day	Census	ICU	Admission			Daily Encounters
Month			Day	Night	Total	
1						
2						
3						
4						
5						
6						
7						
8						
9						
10						
11						
12						
13						
14						
15						
16						
17						
18						
19						
20						
21						
22						
23						
24						
25						
26						
27						
28						
29						
30						
31						

ICU: intensive care unit

for in the medical/surgical units and how many patients were being cared for in the intensive care unit. The next three columns indicate the number of new patients (admissions) that were added to the group's workload—the number admitted during the day, the number admitted at night, and the total number admitted. The last column summarizes the total number of encounters provided by hospitalists for the day.

This census report provides the hospital medicine group with a simple but useful tool for tracking daily hospitalist workload.

Charge Capture System

Charge capture is a vital function within a hospital medicine group. Adequate controls need to be in place to ensure that every patient encounter is identified, properly coded, and submitted to the billing service. An example of a simple charge-capture mechanism used by a hospital medicine group is as follows:

- Upon patient admission, a billing card is created that documents patient demographics, diagnoses, and the Current Procedural Terminology code.
- The card is kept "live" until the patient is discharged from the hospital.
  - o Note: During the patient stay, hospitalists either keep the billing cards in their pockets or keep them in bins dedicated to each hospitalist in the office.
  - o Note: For patients with an extended length of stay, the cards should be retired after one week and new cards created.
- When the patient is discharged, the cards are deposited in a bin or outbox.
- The cards are picked up daily by a courier who works for the billing service.

PCP Communication System

Two-way communication with the patient's PCP is also a critical information system activity for a hospital medicine group, and it is discussed in detail in Chapter 9. The key elements of an effective PCP communication system are as follows:

- Control mechanisms to ensure that the H&P and discharge summary are sent
- Standardized templates for the hospital medicine group
- A close working relationship with the hospital medical records department
- Stat transcription and facsimile services
- Office staff contacts in the PCP office who are familiar with the need to fax key patient information to the hospitalists
- Protocols for when a phone call to the PCP is appropriate

SOPHISTICATED HOSPITALIST INFORMATION SYSTEMS

There are two categories of information system leaders in hospital medicine. The first is made up of hospitalist management companies—regional and national corporations that operate hospital medicine practices in multiple locations. A number of these organizations have developed and implemented sophisticated information systems to support their practice models. The second category of information system leader is composed of software vendors that have targeted the hospitalist market segment. These vendors market and support comprehensive technology solutions for hospital medicine groups.[1]

Following is a list of some of the features and functions of sophisticated software solutions for hospitalists:

1. Allows use of handheld devices and/or laptop computers with Internet access to
   - Collect/enter administrative and clinical data
   - Capture charges (including automated documentation guidelines)
   - Transcribe dictated reports using voice-recognition software
   - Write electronic prescriptions
   - Display patient clinical information (including test results)
   - Access clinical guidelines
   - Access medical knowledge databases
   - Communicate with other hospitalists and community physicians
2. Generates outputs, including
   - H&P document
   - Discharge summary
   - Workload statistics
   - Patient information
   - Quality metrics
3. Integrates with external systems, specifically
   - Hospital information system(s)
   - Billing service system

CONCLUSION

A hospitalist practice combines characteristics of a physician group practice with characteristics of a hospital department. Information systems must support both operational processes and performance reporting. Hospital leaders should recognize that they need to invest in an information infrastructure that may involve manual processes, integration with other hospital systems, and potentially stand-alone vendor software products.

NOTE

1. Information system profiles submitted by hospitalist software vendors to SHM, July 2006.

REFERENCE

Goldsholl, S. 2006. "The Hospitalist Dashboard: A Case Study in the Power of Data." Presentation for the Society of Hospital Medicine's Practice Management course.

CHAPTER 17

Hospitalist Billing and Revenue

Key Message

- Hospitalist compensation should include production-based incentives.
- Hospitalists should engage a billing service that is familiar with hospitalists.
- Billing should be built into the day-to-day operations of the practice.

Billing and revenue generation are often overlooked and underaddressed issues for hospitalist programs. Hospital executives and hospitalist medical directors often focus on minimizing the expense associated with operating their hospitalist program, without realizing that opportunities are available to increase revenue. As with any economic enterprise, revenue generation must be a priority.

A hospital executive should understand the following three principles when addressing the billing and revenue issues for hospitalists:

1. Hospitalist compensation should include production-based incentives.
2. Hospitalists should engage a billing service that is familiar with hospitalists.

3. Billing should be built into the day-to-day operations of the practice.

Also, hospital executives should be aware that hospitalists may have different billing patterns than community physicians who spend most of their time in the office, coming to the hospital for short periods to treat their inpatients. Because hospitalists are in the hospital throughout the day, they may spend more time with patients and their families, consulting physicians, nursing staff, and other healthcare professionals in the inpatient environment. As a result, hospitalists may deliver a more intensive level of service. These differences must, of course, be documented. But it means that hospitalists can receive a higher level of reimbursement for the services they render.

PRODUCTION-BASED INCENTIVES

A significant proportion of hospitalists are employees, typically of hospitals or medical schools. There is the potential (even a likelihood) in these employed environments that the hospitalists do not develop an ownership mentality. In a pure salaried environment, the billing revenue generated by the individual hospitalist and the practice in total would not directly affect the pocketbook of the hospitalist. As might be expected, this environment is not likely to lead to a commitment to maximize billing revenue. Revenue could be lost from some or all of the following sources:

- *Lost charges.* The hospitalist does not identify or bill for all of the services performed.
- *Inadequate documentation.* The hospitalist does not document the full extent of services performed.
- *Undercoding.* The hospitalist assigns a billing code that does not reflect the services performed.
- *Inadequate collections.* The billing service neglects to follow up on health plan denials for hospitalist billings, and the hospitalists

themselves may have little incentive and/or interest in addressing the problem.

An effective strategy for avoiding these problems and maximizing billing revenue for hospitalists is to implement production-based incentive compensation. This can be combined with quality-based incentives, when appropriate. (See Chapter 13 for a more detailed discussion of hospitalist compensation.) A variety of production incentive schemes can be used that incorporate the following elements:

- *Basis of the incentive.* This can include work relative value units (wRVUs), encounters, admissions, billed charges, collections, or some combination of these metrics.
- *Incentive threshold.* Below this amount, the hospitalist does not receive any incentive; above this amount, the hospitalist shares in the additional production.
- *Amount of incentive.* The incentive has to have some substance to affect the behavior of the hospitalist; an impact of at least 10 percent is recommended.

Survey data (see Table 17.1) from Society of Hospital Medicine (2006) examined hospitalists under three different compensation models: pure salary (28 percent), a mix of salary and incentives (67 percent), and pure production-based compensation (5 percent). As is shown by the data, the stronger the incentives, the greater the production by hospitalists.

BILLING SERVICE

Hospitalists should expect the billing service to be actively involved in their hospitalist practice. Billing service staff should conduct regular training sessions, educating the hospitalists on the documentation and coding requirements for the types of encounters and

Table 17.1. Production by Compensation Model

	Median wRVUs	Median Encounters	Median Billed Charges*
Salary	2,824	1,998	$276,000
Mix of salary and incentives	3,321	2,404	$333,000
Pure production-based compensation	4,451	2,829	$392,000
All hospitalists	3,213	2,328	$324,000

* See Table 4.1 for median charges per hospitalist broken out by region, experience, specialty, and employment model.
Source: SHM (2006).

procedures performed by the hospitalists. They should be available by phone to answer coding and documentation questions from hospitalists. In addition, they should conduct periodic audits of the hospitalists' charts to determine if they are sufficiently documenting and assigning appropriate codes based on the documentation.

The billing service should provide regular reports. The reports should be hospitalist specific and should allow each hospitalist to determine how he is performing compared to others in the practice and with regard to any production-based compensation program. Figures 17.1 and 17.2 illustrate sample wRVU reports for an individual hospitalist. Similar reports should be generated for other production measures (encounters, admissions, billed charges, collections), as well as reports that compare the billing patterns of the hospitalists in the practice, providing a summary of production for the entire group.

Finally, the billing service should be aggressive and active in pursuing collections from health plans and public payers. Insurers may not be aware that the submitted claims are from hospitalists or that hospitalists might have different practice patterns from office-based

Figure 17.1. Year-to-Date Summary of wRVUs Generated

	wRVUs: Month	wRVUs: YTD
January		
February		
March		
April		
May		
June		
July		
August		
September		
October		
November		
December		
Total		

physicians. The billing service should make an effort to educate the payer and pursue denied claims.

PRACTICE OPERATIONS

Billing requirements need to be thoroughly integrated with the day-to-day operations of a hospitalist practice. A charge capture process needs to become a routine part of the practice activities. At one extreme are simple manual and paper-based systems that can be implemented. For example, the hospitalist can create an index card for each admission and record the services rendered. If the length of stay becomes longer than the norm, the index card could be submitted and a second card created. At the other extreme, the practice can implement an electronic charge capture system, using hand-held technology (see the discussion in Chapter 16).

Figure 17.2. Current Month Detail of wRVUs Generated

Code	Current Month			Year to Date		
	#	%	wRVUs	#	%	wRVUs
Admission: 99221						
Admission: 99222						
Admission: 99223						
Subsequent visit: 99231						
Subsequent visit: 99232						
Subsequent visit: 99233						
Discharge: 99238						
Discharge: 99239						
Consult: 99251						
Consult: 99252						
Consult: 99253						
Consult: 99254						
Consult: 99255						
Critical care: 99291						
Critical care: 99291						
Other codes						
Total						

Note: Percentages are computed in category (i.e., sum % for 99221, 222, 223, etc. = 100%).

A hospitalist practice also needs administrative support to address the billing process. An administrative staff person should be responsible for knowing all of the patients on the hospitalists' census and ensuring that charge data are received from those hospitalists who are actively treating patients. The staff person should also be the point of contact with the billing service, making sure that the billing information is submitted in a timely fashion. The staff person serves a vital control function in the billing process.

Finally, the practice needs to incorporate billing and revenue status and review meetings into its schedule. At a minimum, hospitalists should meet quarterly to review production, both at the individual hospitalist level and at the overall group level. The meetings should include a representative from the billing service and the administrative staff person. These meetings present an opportunity to discuss and resolve problems and to review the potential impact of the incentive program on hospitalist compensation.

CONCLUSION

A hospital medicine group should be run in a businesslike manner. Maximizing billing revenue must be a priority for successful hospitalist practices. This chapter outlines a series of recommendations with regard to incentives, the role and responsibilities of a billing service, reporting, and operational processes that can improve the billing revenue for hospitalists.

REFERENCE

Society of Hospital Medicine (SHM). 2006. *2005–2006 SHM Survey: State of the Hospital Medicine Movement.* Philadelphia, PA: Society of Hospital Medicine.

CHAPTER 18

Practice Management Issues in Pediatric Hospitalist Programs[1]

Key Message	The activities of a pediatric hospitalist program vary significantly, depending on the hospital environment. The return on investment for pediatric programs is typically more difficult to justify than for adult hospitalist programs.

According to survey data from Society of Hospital Medicine (SHM 2006), 8 to 10 percent of all hospitalists are pediatricians. Pediatric hospitalist programs present some unique issues for hospital executives and hospitalist leaders. This chapter discusses the following topics:

- What pediatric hospitalist programs do
- Economic considerations
- Scheduling and staffing issues
- Compensation and incentives
- Billing and coding
- Use of nurse practitioners and physician assistants
- Other considerations

PEDIATRIC HOSPITALIST PROGRAMS: WHAT THEY DO

Pediatric hospitalist programs can vary significantly depending on the needs of the community and the services provided by the institution. For example, in a tertiary care academic children's hospital, pediatric hospitalist programs often provide attending coverage for a teaching service on the general pediatric wards during regular daytime hours. Residents provide in-house after-hours coverage with attending support on-call from home. A hospitalist-run nonteaching service may also be in place. Hospitalist participation in the emergency department (ED) is limited to accepting admissions, and involvement in the pediatric intensive care unit (PICU) is limited to patient transfers. Pediatric hospitalists have minimal if any involvement with the neonatal intensive care unit (NICU). Hospitalists may or may not provide well-newborn care. Increasingly, surgeons and pediatric subspecialists may request hospitalist comanagement or consultation, but given their formal pediatric subspecialty training, many pediatric subspecialists and surgeons manage some of their patients by themselves. Expert pediatric nurses perform IV, venipuncture, and other procedural services. Full-time, exclusively pediatric staff provide nursing education, respiratory therapy, speech therapy, occupational therapy, pharmacy, case management, child life, quality improvement, patient safety, and other associated pediatric support services.

Contrast this to a medium-sized community hospital. It may have a small, separate pediatric ward that occasionally houses adults when a bed shortage exists on the adult units and pediatrics has vacancies. The hospitalist may need to place many of the IVs and perform the difficult venipunctures. Adult emergency medicine physicians may staff the ED without any pediatric emergency medicine support. If the ED needs a pediatric consult, the hospitalist is called. A general surgeon may feel comfortable performing an appendectomy on a 14-year-old, but the surgeon may need a pediatric consultation for an 8-year-old. Radiology staff may not be comfortable performing certain studies on smaller pediatric patients. Continuous albuterol therapy for pediatric patients with severe asthma may exceed the nursing and/or monitoring resources and policies of the general pediatric unit. A neonatologist may cover cesarean section and other high-risk deliveries during the day, but a hospitalist may provide coverage at night.

ECONOMICS OF PEDIATRIC HOSPITALIST PROGRAMS

Pediatric reimbursement patterns are different from adult-unit reimbursement patterns. Many pediatric patients have Medicaid coverage, and Medicaid typically reimburses considerably less than Medicare. This significantly affects the economics of pediatric general inpatient care. Furthermore, pediatric inpatient care is intrinsically more time consuming than adult inpatient care. Every pediatric inpatient visit involves some form of a family conference; the physician is always talking with the parent in addition to the child patient. Routine communication simply requires more time. Careful coding can capture some of this activity by documenting counseling time and adding multiple visits throughout the day into one higher-level code, but services continue to be poorly reimbursed. Procedures (IV, venipunctures, catheterization) take longer for pediatric patients than for adults because of parental concern, lack of patient cooperation, and smaller size.

The return on investment (ROI) analysis for a pediatric hospitalist program should take a broad view of the value-added calculation. Similar to adult hospitalist programs, published research supports average length of stay and cost savings in the 5 to 15 percent range (Landrigan et al. 2006). However, pediatric reimbursement may be based on per diems, not diagnosis-related groups or case rates. If hospitalists reduce lengths of stay by eliminating the latter days of a patient's stay when costs per day are lower, the net economic impact may be negative for the hospital. However, in the long run and for most payers and contracts, the hospital will end up benefiting financially by providing more efficient and lower-cost services.

Pediatric lengths of stay are significantly affected by how psychologically and materially prepared a family is to provide ongoing care at home. Because of language barriers, socioeconomic considerations, cultural differences, and limited outpatient resources, discharge is often delayed for reasons outside of the hospitalist's control. Nonetheless, a well-run hospitalist program should be able to identify these cases and reduce extended stays by initiating early discharge planning. These difficulties will not disappear with initiation of a hospitalist program, but within one institution the mix should not differ significantly across hospitalists. Comparisons from one institution to another should be made more carefully. These interinstitutional comparisons are useful for identifying systems issues to improve within a hospital but are less useful for identifying inefficiencies in individual providers.

Pediatric hospitalists provide other system benefits that may be more difficult to measure from a financial perspective. Consider the following examples:

- If a hospitalist was not available for a difficult IV placement, the IV team, the anesthesiologist, or the pediatrician on call at home would be called.
- The availability of a pediatric hospitalist may encourage more subspecialists and surgeons to provide inpatient pediatric care at a community hospital, resulting in an increased volume and a financially more attractive case mix.
- Primary care physicians may refer more patients to a hospital that offers quality pediatric hospitalist services (although many pediatricians will still choose to come to the hospital on a daily basis to visit their newborns).
- In a tertiary care children's hospital, pediatric hospitalists may increase the efficiency of pediatric surgeons and subspecialists, resulting in reduced wait times, improved access, better quality, and increased revenue.

- Increased throughput on the pediatric ward can help decompress the PICU and ED, thereby increasing capacity.

Pediatric hospitalists also contribute to improved quality of care. In the community hospital setting, the hospitalists (and in particular the hospital medicine group leader) are often advocates for pediatrics within the entire hospital, addressing the following roles:

- Driving the institution's pediatric quality improvement efforts
- Serving on the pediatric rapid response team
- Caring for the uninsured
- Implementing a pediatric patient safety program
- Interfacing with the ED if no pediatric emergency physician is available
- Developing clinical pathways
- Providing the bulk of the inpatient care measured by publicly reported (or pay for performance) pediatric indicators that are likely to be implemented

It is this broad view of the value of a pediatric hospital medicine program that is the most compelling economic argument for pediatric hospitalists. While rigorous financial calculations are generally missing, the move of such global organizations as Kaiser Permanente and other integrated systems to the pediatric hospitalist programs suggests that significant overall value and efficiencies can be achieved in the hospitalist model.

Almost all pediatric hospitalist programs require financial support. Benchmark data are not available, but estimates range from 25 percent to 50 percent of the cost of the program, or potentially more depending on payer mix. However, the need to subsidize a pediatric hospitalist program may create a significant financial challenge for smaller institutions. A pediatric hospitalist program is not the right choice for all institutions.

One option is to gradually introduce a program with one full-time equivalent pediatric hospitalist who provides limited inpatient coverage and ED support. Most primary care pediatricians and family practitioners in the community would still do some of their own inpatient care. The benefits and economic reality of the hospitalist program can be evaluated without undermining the infrastructure of current pediatric inpatient activity.

SCHEDULING AND STAFFING

Schedules and staffing models for pediatric hospital medicine programs vary significantly depending on the services provided and the hospital environment. Programs that provide delivery room coverage typically need 24/7 in-house presence. Academic programs generally have built-in night coverage from house staff. Programs that focus on inpatient care will benefit from continuity of care on the inpatient service by having a single hospitalist work longer periods of time in a row on the inpatient service (e.g., 4 to 28 days). Continuity is less of a concern for programs that place more emphasis on ED services, delivery room coverage, or after-hours coverage of the NICU or PICU. If night-time volume is not excessive, 16-hour overnight shifts (or even 24-hour shifts) can be useful in these settings as this provides continuity of care over a 16- to 24-hour period and allows direct sign-out from the intensivist or neonatologist to the hospitalist covering at night rather than indirect sign-out from the daytime hospitalist.

Workloads for pediatric hospitalist programs should be sufficient to allow two visits daily for most patients to promote prompt responses to laboratory tests and changes in the patient's condition and to update parents and answer questions. When workloads limit hospitalists to one visit per patient per day, afternoon and evening discharge opportunities are lost and length of stay and costs will increase, undermining the economic benefits of the hospitalist model. A limit of 15 to 20 encounters per physician per day is a good starting point when planning physician staffing levels and workload. Procedures should be counted as an encounter, and extended repeat follow-up visits the same day should also be counted as a separate encounter from the morning visit.

The staffing and scheduling considerations outlined in chapters 10 and 11 can be applied to pediatric hospitalist programs. Because pediatric hospital medicine programs are typically smaller than adult programs, few opportunities arise for economies of scale. Generally one is trying to decide between zero and one physician in-house at night (i.e., on call from home versus in-house call), and one to two or two to three physicians in-house during the daytime. When combined with the problem of covering multiple geographic and functional areas of the hospital, efficient staffing becomes challenging. Furthermore, pediatric inpatient admission rates vary significantly throughout the year, particularly in community hospitals. Winter volumes are much higher than summer volumes. Schedules can be designed to take advantage of this variation by concentrating vacation time in the summer and reducing summer staffing levels. Some programs even hire "winterist" physicians.

COMPENSATION AND INCENTIVES

A relatively uniform standard for pediatric hospitalists is to work 40 to 48 hours per week for 47 weeks per year (four weeks are allowed for paid time off, one week for continuing medical education). Experience proves this to be a sustainable schedule, depending on the amount of night and weekend work. Few pediatric programs work a 7-on/7-off schedule, although academic programs often have relatively infrequent more intensive periods when the physician is on service, with 60- to 80-hour weeks being common.

Pediatric hospitalist compensation varies by job description, duties, and workload. The latest SHM (2006) compensation figures report a median salary of $139,000 and mean salary of $146,000 (n = 261). Note that pediatric compensation is lower than adult compensation in part because of the higher proportion of pediatric hospitalists employed in academic settings. Much variation occurs among pediatric programs; practices are well served by comparing compensation to other local pediatric hospitalist programs and/or programs with similar job descriptions. Local moonlighting rates can also serve as a useful starting point. Finally, another benchmark is the compensation for an office-based pediatrician in the community. Hospitalists generally are paid at the level of an established general pediatrician in an office practice or a pediatrician working in an urgent-care–type setting, and less than subspecialists. Adjustments should be made for night and weekend coverage.

Incentives are a useful component of pediatric hospitalist compensation but are generally underutilized. Rudimentary pediatric information systems and limited benchmark data discourage the adoption of incentive systems. Pediatrics is not subject to the reporting requirements of the Centers for Medicare and Medicaid Services. Therefore, fewer resources are devoted to developing the requisite infrastructure. Nonetheless, within an institution a practice should be able to modify the adult structure for appropriate pediatric content.

Productivity incentives for pediatricians are complicated by the absence of reimbursement for certain critical and often time-consuming pediatric services. For example, IV insertion can frequently take 60 minutes and may not be reimbursed. Some families require extensive consultation. It is important to track these services, even if the payers do not reimburse them, to understand the full range of services the pediatric hospital medicine program is providing. If the hospitalists were not doing this, someone else would be. Productivity incentives based on a percentage of charges rather than collections may be appropriate. This eliminates disincentives based on payer mix, collection rates, or the refusal of insurance companies to recognize certain codes. In fact, some pediatric hospitalist programs create internal codes with internally agreed-upon value units to track services the program values (e.g., curbside consults, assisting nurses with procedures). These services are tallied by the billing software to track performance, but no bill is submitted to an insurance company. Incorporating these internal codes into the billing paperwork encourages hospitalists to actively track their total productivity. When translating charges into a financial incentive program, simply adjusting the percentage modifier down from percentage charges or collections is enough to create an effective incentive program. Generally, Medicare billing guidelines and Stark law regulations apply equally to Medicaid and other pediatric services.

Many pediatric hospitalist programs choose to use internal, program-specific quality markers as the basis of incentive compensation that rewards performance. Examples include committee participation, parent satisfaction, coding accuracy, communication promptness and completeness, and pathway adherence. Given the absence of identified national standards in pediatrics and limited benchmarks, these markers of quality may be the most effective incentives.

BILLING AND CODING

Current Procedural Terminology (CPT) coding for pediatrics does not differ significantly from adults with the exception of global critical care codes for both neonatal and pediatric critical care. If hospitalists provide after-hours coverage in the NICU or PICU, a portion of the global fee received by the neonatologist or pediatric intensivist is intended to support after-hours coverage. This revenue, which is typically lost to the hospitalist program, should be considered part of the value-added calculation. Given the shortage of pediatric intensivists (and other pediatric specialists), one may view hospitalists as a recruiting tool or cost for intensivists.

Pediatric hospitalists should be knowledgeable about documentation and coding requirements. In particular, efforts should be made to capture the additional reimbursement available that comes from multiple visits throughout the course of the day. This requires physicians to chart frequently. Electronic and in particular handheld data-capture systems that require submission of a CPT code with each note may be beneficial.

Observation codes are a frequent conundrum for pediatric hospitalists. Standards vary widely across states, institutions, and payers. Generally, the hospitalist should bill consistently with the hospital to avoid rejections. Hospital reimbursement will exceed physician reimbursement and should drive the overall billing policy. If hospitalists are under-reimbursed for observation-level services, this should be addressed in the subsidy for the ROI calculation.

USE OF MID-LEVEL PRACTITIONERS

Nurse practitioners (NPs) and physician assistants (PAs) can be very effective members of the pediatric hospital medicine team. Generally, they work best in a focused capacity under a physician's supervision in groups that have a consistent style, both clinically and logistically. If NPs and PAs are an accepted part of office practice in the community, they are likely to be welcomed in the inpatient arena. When the hospitalist job description requires multitasking across multiple venues, it is frequently more efficient to base the NP/PA in one particular unit where he has developed expertise, and rely on the hospitalist to multitask.

ORGANIZATIONAL RESOURCES FOR PEDIATRIC HOSPITALISTS

Although this chapter has emphasized the variations from one program to another, core activities are shared among them as well, and pediatric hospitalists benefit significantly from networking with each other and with adult hospitalists. The logistic and management expertise available through SHM is crucial to any pediatric hospital medicine group leader and is a strong motivator for career-oriented pediatric hospitalists. Other key resources for pediatric hospitalists are listed in Table 18.1. Given the range of pediatric hospital medicine programs, it is helpful to be able to network with programs of similar scope.

SHM, the American Academy of Pediatrics, and the American Pediatric Association cosponsor an annual pediatric hospital meeting each summer that provides an invaluable forum for pediatric hospitalists.

Table 18.1. Organizational Resources for Pediatric Hospitalists

Organization	Resources	Web Address
Society of Hospital Medicine, Pediatric Committee	Logistical and operational issues for hospital medicine programs, employment opportunities, leadership training	www.hospital medicine.org
American Academy of Pediatrics, Section on Hospital Medicine	Clinical materials, child advocacy, employment opportunities	www.aap.org
Pediatric Hospital Medicine, listserv	Open forum for all pediatric hospital medicine issues	www.aap.org/ sections/ hospcare
Ambulatory Pediatric Association, Hospital Medicine Special Interest Group	Academic pediatric hospital medicine, research and teaching, home of Pediatric Research in Inpatient Settings network	www.ambpeds.org
National Institute for Children's Healthcare Quality	Focus on children's healthcare quality	www.NICHQ.org

OTHER CONSIDERATIONS

Recommendations regarding the recruitment and retention of hospitalists provided in Chapter 7 also apply to pediatric hospitalists. Successful programs will experience low turnover and will be able to rely on word of mouth for recruitment, especially if they are located near a training program. Print and electronic services for job advertising are available.

Consultants may be helpful in designing a new program, but few "off the shelf" models are available in pediatrics. Some companies that provide outsourced neonatology and pediatric critical care services to hospitals have recently branched out into hospitalist services. Most pediatric hospitalists are employees of an academic center, a hospital, or a local multispecialty medical group. There are few private-practice pediatric hospitalists.

The key qualifications for a pediatric hospitalist are enthusiasm for inpatient pediatrics, effective communication skills, completion of residency training, and current pediatric advanced life-support certification. Academic hospitalists will benefit from formal fellowship training to develop research and teaching skills, but this is not required for the general pediatric hospitalist. Subspecialists who function as hospitalists can provide additional expertise but should wear a generalist hat in most of their hospitalist medicine work.

When establishing a pediatric hospital medicine program, organizations must ensure appropriate outpatient follow-up of children with no or limited access to care. The hospital medicine group can assume this responsibility on an inpatient basis; some other entity must be available for outpatient services, such as a clinic associated with the hospital. Another option is to have the community pediatricians responsible for initial outpatient follow-up for any patient admitted to the hospitalist service the day they are on call.

CONCLUSION

A pediatric hospitalist program will not resolve all the pediatric concerns for a community hospital. For most community hospitals, the hospitalists will become pediatric advocates and representatives on appropriate hospital committees and improvement efforts. However, additional expertise, insights, and political capital will be needed to create systemwide change in such parts of the hospital as nursing, respiratory therapy, case management, radiology, lab services, pharmacy, and the ED. Do not expect the hospitalist to be able to do it all. Do expect the hospitalist to work with leaders within each of these areas to advocate for pediatrics within the hospital.

NOTE

1. Jack Percelay, M.D., contributed material to this chapter.

REFERENCES

Landrigan, C. P., P. H. Conway, S. Edwards, and R. Srivastava. 2006. "Pediatric Hospitalists: A Systematic Review of the Literature." *Pediatrics* 117 (5): 1736–44.

Society of Hospital Medicine (SHM). 2006. *2005–2006 SHM Survey: State of the Hospital Medicine Movement*. Philadelphia, PA: Society of Hospital Medicine.

Differences in Hospitalist Practice Management Issues, by Organizational Model

As mentioned in Chapter 2, approximately 2,500 hospital medicine groups exist in the United States. These groups can be categorized under five models. The major characteristics of each of these models are described in Chapter 2. This appendix presents a comparison of these models across 11 key practice management issues.

Appendix A. Differences in Hospitalist Practice Management Issues, by Organizational Model

	Hospital or Hospital-Owned Corporation (33%)	Academic Institution (20%)	Multispecialty/Primary Care Medical Group (14%)	Local Hospitalist-Only Group (12%)	Multistate Hospitalist-Only Group/Management Company (19%)
Organization-Specific Issues	• Pressures (re: efficiency; e.g., LOS) • Pressures (re: quality) • Medical staff perceptions (re: hospitalists) • Nurse retention • Throughput • Joint Commission review • Surgical comanagement	• Same as hospital employed • Teaching • Research • Resident work limitations • Community medicine	• Partner-to-partner interactions • Revenue generation • Efficiency • Access to office practice • Managed care contracts/capitation	• Revenue generation • Growth/marketing • Service quality	• Same as local hospitalist-only group • Need to build a formal, replicable infrastructure (e.g., training, operations)
Hospital Financial Support	• Driven by hospital administration	• Same as hospital employed	• Relevant only if hospital asks group for services (e.g., unassigned patients)	• Relevant only if hospital asks group for services (e.g., unassigned patients)	• Depends on model—some are independent groups and some are a contracted service by the hospital

Hospitalist Recruitment	• Driven by growth of patient volume • Retention is a challenge • Per SHM survey, this model employs more nurse practitioners and physician assistants	• Driven by growth of patient volume • Retention is a challenge • In-house source of physicians (graduates) • Per SHM survey, many academic programs are pediatric	• Driven by growth of patient volume • Retention is a challenge • In-house source of physicians (partners)	• Driven by growth of patient volume • Retention is a challenge	• Driven by growth of patient volume of a local practice • Retention is a challenge • National challenge as new clients/locations are added
Staffing Model	Per SHM survey: • 60% shift based • 15% call based • 25% mixed	Per SHM survey: • 24% shift based • 23% call based • 53% mixed	Per SHM survey: • 34% shift based • 25% call based • 42% mixed	Per SHM survey: • 46% shift based • 35% call based • 20% mixed	Per SHM survey: • 20% shift based • 41% call based • 39% mixed

Continued ...

	Hospital or Hospital-Owned Corporation (33%)	Academic Institution (20%)	Multispecialty/Primary Care Medical Group (14%)	Local Hospitalist-Only Group (12%)	Multistate Hospitalist-Only Group/Management Company (19%)
Compensation	Per SHM survey: • 28% all salary • 3% all productivity • 68% mixed Median: $172,000	Per SHM survey: • 44% all salary • 0% all productivity • 56% mixed Median: $150,000	Per SHM survey: • 29% all salary • 10% all productivity • 60% mixed Median: $178,000	Per SHM survey: • 22% all salary • 11% all productivity • 65% mixed Median: $166,000	Per SHM survey: • 7% all salary • 0% all productivity • 93% mixed Median: $168,000
Medical Director	• Hospital employee	• Medical school/hospital employee	• Member of group's internal medicine department	• Often the founder of the group	• Member of senior management • Clinical leader
Billing Issues	• Often overlooked • Performed by hospital or vendors chosen by hospital	• Same as hospital employed	• Core competency (although not necessarily for hospitalist services)	• Core competency	• Core competency (often centralized)

Systems and Information Technology	• Often manual or phone based • Need hospital IT integration for reports	• Same as hospital employed	• "Piggyback" on the multispecialty group's system	• Acquire practice management software or billing vendor	• Often major investment in IT (more than billing)
Marketing Issues	• Typically passive marketing to new PCPs	• Same as hospital employed	• Not relevant, unless to other medical groups	• *Critical* to key customers (e.g., hospitals, physicians, payers)	• *Critical* to key customers (e.g., hospitals, physicians, payers)
Challenges and Risks	• Staffing models • Sufficient funding • Proving value • Payer mix • Billing/collections	• Same as hospital employed • Limited payments for research/teaching	• Partner dissatisfaction (e.g., re: economics, service) • Achieving group consensus on model	• Managing/financing growth • Payer reimbursement • Contracts	• Same as local hospitalist-only group • Investments in infrastructure

LOS: length of stay; IT: information technology; PCP: primary care physician

Note: Percentages do not always add up to 100%, either because of rounding or because of the exclusion of the "other" categories.

Source: SHM (2006).

Recommendations for Recruiting Hospitalists

The two most important keys to a successful ongoing hospitalist recruitment plan are as follows:

1. Always be on the lookout for internists (or pediatricians or family physicians) in traditional practice in the hospital's service area who might be interested in becoming hospitalists.
2. Build a strong, ongoing relationship with the residents at the closest internal medicine (or pediatrics or family practice) training program.

RECRUITMENT OF LOCAL PHYSICIANS— SUGGESTIONS

1. Keep an eye open for relatively new physicians (i.e., in practice three years or less) in the community who do not have a "mature" outpatient practice and, if qualified, ask them if they want to join the hospitalist practice.
2. Encourage hospitalists to actively participate in local or statewide medical societies and meetings where they might meet potential hospitalists.

3. Ask doctors in all specialties at your institution to identify friends or acquaintances who might be candidates for the practice (e.g., people from their own training program).
4. Call local public health departments and clinics to let physicians know you have hospitalist openings.
5. If a member of a local primary care practice wishes to become a hospitalist, consider offering recruitment assistance to the primary care group to replace the doctor.

RECRUITMENT FROM A NEARBY TRAINING PROGRAM—SUGGESTIONS

1. Host a dinner for second- and third-year residents at a nice restaurant near the residency program a couple of times each year. In addition to hospitalists, a few members of the hospital's administrative and medical staff should attend the dinner. This is worthwhile even if the training program is several hours away from your hospital.
2. Establish a good contact person at the nearby training program(s). Often, the chief resident (rather than the program director) can be most effective in identifying potential candidates and arranging dinners. Also, take advantage of existing relationships that any of the hospital's doctors might have with people in the residency program (either residents or faculty). If you are successful in recruiting a resident as a hospitalist, she might help to recruit friends and former colleagues from the residency program.
3. Offer to financially sponsor one or more appropriate resident activities—such as funding a research grant or sponsoring a resident to attend a Society of Hospital Medicine (SHM) event or other hospital medicine–related conferences.
4. Offer to have those hospitalists with good public speaking skills give didactic lectures on topics related to hospital medicine at the training program's conferences.

5. Consider offering an elective "away" rotation for residents to spend a month working with the hospitalists at your hospital. This is an effective recruiting tool but requires a lot of work to set up.
6. Offer to participate in other activities that would give practicing hospitalists face time with the residents.

If recruiting mid-level practitioners from training programs, these approaches can be adopted for physician assistants or nurse practitioners in training.

RECRUITING FOR A START-UP PRACTICE

Many new practices have found success by initially recruiting hospitalists from the local physician community. The benefit is that you are familiar with the quality of the doctor's work. And because he has already developed a connection to the community, you face a much lower risk that the doctor will leave the practice simply due to unhappiness with living in the community. Furthermore, since other doctors will already know, and presumably think well of this first hospitalist, they are likely to be more forgiving of any initial problems or mistakes as the practice gets up and running. Finally, hiring a local physician saves money on travel and moving expenses.

Institutions developing a new hospitalist practice often wonder if most or all of the initial doctors should have significant postresidency experience, and more specifically, direct experience as a hospitalist. While such experience is desirable, it is not critical. As the hospital medicine movement has grown over the last ten years, many successful hospitalist practices have started with doctors just out of residency. Start with at least one or two doctors with prior experience, but if your only realistic option is to solely start with doctors right out of residency training, it is still reasonable to move ahead. If you start up without experienced hospitalists, you should identify at least one senior member of the hospital's medical staff to serve as a champion and advisor for the new hospitalists for the first year or two.

OTHER RECOMMENDATIONS

1. Encourage all hospitalists to join the SHM. Send at least one hospitalist to the SHM annual meeting every year to build program visibility and relationships.
2. Send out an annual mailing to all of the internal medicine training programs across the country (late fall or winter is the best time).
3. Consider developing relationships with one or more of the physician search firms that work with hospitalist practices. Thus, if you need to use their services, they will already be familiar with your program and needs and can hit the ground running. They may also send you unsolicited resumes. You can get an idea of which firms are active in hospitalist recruitment by looking at the classified ads in the back of publications such as *The Hospitalist* and *Today's Hospitalist*.
4. Post positions in the SHM publications and career center website. The SHM career center is the only Internet-based job site focused solely on hospitalists (see www.hospitalmedicine.org/careercenter). Journals such as the *New England Journal of Medicine* and *Annals of Internal Medicine* are also good places for classified ads.

CONCLUSION

Hospitalist recruitment should be an ongoing priority for most hospital medicine groups. Most hospital medicine groups are likely to experience one or more of the following pressures, which may require adding more hospitalists: (1) greater patient volume, (2) broader responsibilities, and (3) hospitalist turnover.

Sample Hospitalist Practice Brochure

A sample hospitalist program brochure appears on the following pages. As mentioned in chapters 5 and 9, a printed brochure introduces patients to the individual doctors in the program. A brochure, such as the one shown here, also provides an opportunity for the hospital to describe the concept of hospitalist practice.

As this example shows, a hospitalist brochure includes the following elements:

- An explanation of the function and benefits of a hospitalist, in a question-and-answer format
- A short evaluation form, backed by a postage-paid stamp for convenient mailing
- A brief list of the hospitalists in the program

Including a picture of each hospitalist in the brochure helps to familiarize patients to these professionals.

Community General Hospitalist Practice

You have been referred to a Community General physician known as a **hospitalist**.

Hospitalists are doctors who devote their practice to the care of hospitalized patients. Community General hospitalists are board certified in internal medicine. They see hospitalized patients who have been referred by primary care doctors, emergency room doctors, or other physicians at the hospital. They do not see patients outside the hospital.

COMMUNITY GENERAL HOSPITAL

Who are we?

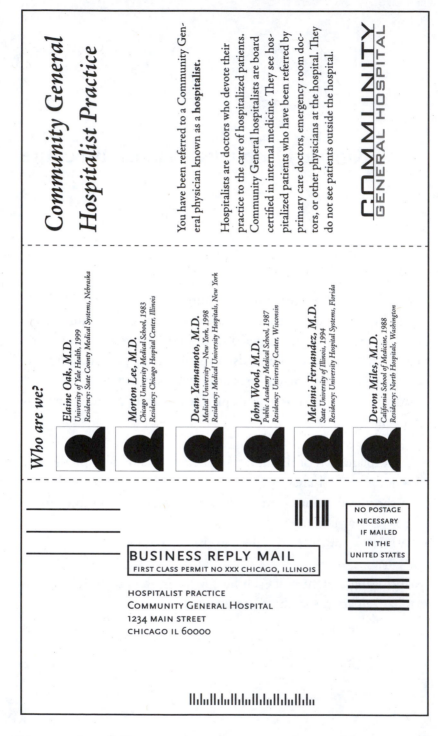

Elaine Oak, M.D.
University of Yale Health, 1999
Residency: State County Medical Systems, Nebraska

Morton Lee, M.D.
Chicago University Medical School, 1983
Residency: Chicago Hospital Center, Illinois

Dean Yamamoto, M.D.
Medical University—New York, 1998
Residency: Medical University Hospitals, New York

John Wood, M.D.
Public Academy Medical School, 1987
Residency: University Center, Wisconsin

Melanie Fernandez, M.D.
State University of Illinois, 1994
Residency: University Hospital Systems, Florida

Devon Miles, M.D.
California School of Medicine, 1988
Residency: North Hospitals, Washington

NO POSTAGE
NECESSARY
IF MAILED
IN THE
UNITED STATES

BUSINESS REPLY MAIL
FIRST CLASS PERMIT NO XXX CHICAGO, ILLINOIS

HOSPITALIST PRACTICE
COMMUNITY GENERAL HOSPITAL
1234 MAIN STREET
CHICAGO IL 60000

☙ Dr. Oak
☙ Dr. Lee
☙ Dr. Yamamoto
☙ Dr. Wood
☙ Dr. Fernandez
☙ Dr. Miles

	Excellent	Very Good	Good	Fair	Poor
Availability of the doctor when needed	5	4	3	2	1
Skill of the doctor(s) treating you	5	4	3	2	1
Courtesy/respect given by the doctor(s)	5	4	3	2	1
Amount of information doctor gave you about your illness and treatment	5	4	3	2	1
Your perception of the doctor's assessment & management of your pain while you were in the hospital	5	4	3	2	1

Why is a hospitalist caring for me?

Your own primary care physician may request that a hospitalist be in charge of your care during the hospital stay. In this way you have the benefit of being seen by a doctor whose practice is entirely focused on the care of hospitalized patients. Additionally, this can enable your primary care doctor to be more available to you in the office, rather than trying to go back and forth between seeing patients in the office and in the hospital.

How does the hospitalist practice work?

The hospitalist will be in charge of your care and will see you every day to direct your treatment while you are in the hospital. This doctor is available to you and your family to answer questions and discuss your care. The hospitalist works at the hospital full-time to provide for your care and attend to any emergencies that may arise. The hospitalist may consult other doctors to participate in your care as well.

The hospitalist will make arrangements for any prescriptions you may need when you are discharged. You may be asked to make an appointment with your primary care doctor or with other doctors soon after discharge.

Since hospitalist do not have an outpatient practice, you will not have an appointment to see the hospitalist again after discharge. You may contact the hospitalist after discharge if you have any questions about the hospital stay.

What is the relationship between the hospitalist and my primary care physician?

The two doctors work together. Your primary care physician can provide information about your past health history to the hospitalists, and the two doctors can discuss any significant findings or events. At the time of your admission and discharge, the hospitalist prepares a detailed report of findings and treatment plans that is sent to your primary care physician.

Your primary care physician asks the hospitalist to be in charge of your care while you are in the hospital, but is welcome to check on you and discuss your care with the hospitalist anytime during your hospital stay. When you are discharged, you will return to the care of your primary care doctor.

What if I need another specialist while in the hospital?

Consultations from other physicians are necessary in some cases, and the hospitalist can arrange for these as necessary. If you have already been seeing other doctors at Community General or elsewhere, be sure to let us know so that we can keep them informed about your hospital stay.

What if I don't have a regular primary care physician?

The Community General hospitalist, and other staff at the hospital, can assist in finding a doctor for you to see after leaving the hospital. Records from your hospital stay can be sent to this physician.

Your feedback is valuable to us. If you have a minute, we would appreciate your opinions about our care. You may give the survey to your nurse or mail it to us at the address on the back of the survey.

How to contact us: If you would like to speak with one of the hospitalists while you or a member of your family is in the hospital, it is best to ask the nurse caring for you to page the doctor. Otherwise you can reach us as follows:
Mailing Address: 1234 Main Street, Chicago, IL 60000
Phone: (555) 123-4567 • Billing Office: (555) 123-456X

Action Steps to Address Hospitalist Career Satisfaction

The five categories of action steps are as follows:

1. Get the facts
2. Organizational/structural strategies
3. Systems strategies
4. Professional development strategies
5. Marketing/relationship strategies

The table on the following pages highlights suggested steps in each category.

Appendix D. Action Steps to Address Hospitalist Career Satisfaction

	Pillar 1 *Reward/Recognition*	Pillar 2 *Workload/Schedule*	Pillar 3 *Control/Autonomy*	Pillar 4 *Community/Environment*
Get the facts	• Conduct a formal review/ analysis of compensation and benefits • Survey medical staff on satisfaction with hospitalists • Survey nursing staff on satisfaction with hospitalists • Survey hospitalists on career satisfaction	• Document hospitalist workload/productivity • Document hospitalist responsibilities • Benchmark workload/ productivity against SHM (2006) survey data • Survey hospitalist perceptions on workload • Research hospitalist scheduling/staffing models	• Use the job-fit questionnaire to profile the control elements of the hospitalist practice • Become familiar with the hospital's leadership and committee structure • Understand key payer issues that might affect inpatient care • Review the hospitalist job description	• Review and communicate hospital policies on harassment and discrimination • Research availability of professional counseling resources • Determine which, if any, hospitalists look at their job as a temporary position
Organizational/ structural strategies	• Create an ownership mentality in the hospitalist group • Implement an incentive compensation program • Establish a formal negotiation process with hospital leadership • Establish a formal negotiation process with medical staff • Change the organizational model (to private group) • Create an organizational structure that recognizes hospitalists' multiple roles	• Implement an incentive compensation program • Add administrative support staff • Add nonphysician staff • Add additional physician staff • Use part-time hospitalists • Use nocturnists • Include dedicated time for nonclinical work in the job definition	• Involve hospitalists in participative decision making on key work-life issues • Create an ownership mentality in the hospitalist group • Establish a formal negotiation process with hospital leadership • Establish a formal negotiation process with medical staff • Establish mission and value statements for the hospitalist group	• Pursue leadership in hospital committees • Conduct regular hospitalist group meetings • Define hospitalist group goals • Create a culture of teamwork and empower members to voice concerns

| Systems strategies | • Create an awards committee to recognize exceptional performance
• Incorporate job satisfaction into quarterly hospitalist reviews | • Implement a new schedule/staffing model (shorter but more shifts? backup call?)
• Generate reports on hospitalist productivity and workload
• Establish backup plan for family/medical emergencies
• Use a dedicated on-call pager (perhaps also covering admissions, rapid response teams)
• Maximize pager technology
• Pool nonurgent nursing concerns
• Use as-needed admission orders | • Document in writing understandings with hospitalists about workload/schedule
• Establish formal agreement with medical staff on types of patients seen by hospitalists
• Seek improvements in hospital processes that affect hospitalist performance (e.g., throughput)
• Establish standards for hospitalist processes (e.g., primary care physician communication, sign out, admission, discharge) | • Structure sufficient time for patient/family communications
• Ensure dedicated time for nonpatient care responsibilities
• Create a mentorship program with regularly scheduled meetings |

Continued ...

	Pillar 1 Reward/Recognition	Pillar 2 Workload/Schedule	Pillar 3 Control/Autonomy	Pillar 4 Community/Environment
Professional development strategies	• Establish peer or individual supervision • Identify and take a proactive role in establishing mentoring relationships • Organize/participate in hospitalist chapter meetings • Clearly set expectations for individual hospitalists • Clarify individual performance goals and acknowledge when they are achieved	• Recognize individual goals/preferences in scheduling/staffing • Clearly describe the group's work philosophy to new hires • Measure and discuss productivity and workload with hospitalists	• Use the job-fit questionnaire to assess potential hospitalists (and share information with the candidates) • Allow hospitalists to choose which committees and/or projects they want to participate on • Establish core values that promulgate peer support and rewards for identifying problems and asking for help • Get leadership training for hospitalist director	• Include hospitalists in key meetings • Develop communication skills via conferences/continuing medical education • Communicate job requirements/expectations to new hires • Establish a journal club • Reimburse membership in SHM and other professional groups • Establish personal goals/expectations • Ensure sufficient vacations to revitalize

Marketing/relationship strategies			
• Formally present performance results to hospital leadership/ medical staff (hospitalist quarterly reports) • Assume responsibility for physician education programs at hospital • Take the hospital CEO on hospitalist rounds • Pursue leadership roles on committees, in teaching, in research, etc. • Establish formal team meetings with nurses, discharge planning, etc. • Pursue public relations opportunities in hospital and community publications • Seek speaking engagements at community, specialty, and national professional meetings • Seek advocates/allies among hospital leadership/ medical staff	• Communicate schedule/ staffing model to hospital leadership • Communicate schedule/ staffing model to medical staff • Work with nurses and other team members on productivity	• Seek representation on hospital committees/ boards that affect hospitalists • Establish formal team meetings with nurses, discharge planning, etc. • Seek advocates/allies among hospital leadership/medical staff	• Conduct meetings with hospital administration to discuss hospitalist performance • Conduct meetings with referring physicians to discuss hospitalist performance • Conduct meetings with nonreferring physicians to market the program • Conduct meetings with specialist physicians to educate them about hospitalists • Conduct meetings with nursing administration • Announce addition of new hospitalists • Create a hospitalist program website for patients, families, and physicians • Print and distribute a hospitalist program brochure

Sample Communication Plan for a Hospitalist Program

COMMUNICATION WITH PRIMARY CARE PHYSICIANS

At Admission

- The emergency department (ED) physician speaks with the referring primary care physician (PCP) (Dr. X). If the decision is to admit, the hospitalist is contacted.
- If possible, the PCP provides the patient with a brochure explaining the hospitalist practice; otherwise, this is done by the hospitalist.
- The hospitalist writes an order in the chart to "Notify Dr. X that the patient has been admitted." When desired by the referring PCP, or as necessary for clinical reasons, the hospitalist may call the referring PCP directly.
- The referring PCP's office is called by the hospitalist or administrative staff person at the hospital and notified of the admission. The staff at the referring PCP's office automatically retrieves the patient's office chart and faxes the most recent records to the hospital to be placed on the chart.

- The hospitalist dictates a history and physical at the time of admission; it is transcribed within hours and faxed to the referring PCP and placed on the inpatient chart.
- The admitting order form completed by the hospitalist provides a checklist of other outside records that are requested by the hospitalist. The hospitalist staff (e.g., rounding assistant) follows up to get these additional outside records.
- Prior inpatient records are made available to the hospitalist in the ED or the hospital unit.
- The hospital makes every effort to identify the referring PCP to facilitate the communication of test results, etc.

During the Inpatient Stay

- The hospitalist and the PCP communicate by telephone only as needed.
- An effort is made to reduce the number of times the hospital staff pages the hospitalist by
  o leaving notes for the hospitalist on a communication sheet in the patient's chart
  o each unit accumulating nonemergent pages and contacting the physician approximately every two hours
  o as much as possible, grouping the inpatient team's patients within the same units

At Discharge

- Hospitalist discharge summaries are dictated, transcribed, and faxed to the referring PCP before the close of business that day (unless discharged late in the day).
- The patient is given a discharge summary when appropriate (e.g., when uncertainty exists surrounding patient's follow-up physician).

- All hospitalists use the same format for discharge summaries to make it easier for PCPs to find pertinent information in the document.
- The hospitalist phones the PCP when necessary or when desired by the PCP.
- The test results pending at discharge and any recommended follow-up evaluations (e.g., check prothrombin time/INR [international normalized ratio]) twice a week until stable in therapeutic range) are highlighted for the PCP in the discharge summary.
- Patients discharged to skilled nursing facilities (SNFs) should have clear notes identifying the responsible physician in the SNF.

COMMUNICATION WITH THE PATIENT, FAMILY, AND HOME CARE PROVIDER

- The hospitalist describes the hospitalist–referring PCP partnership to patient and family.
- A hospitalist brochure is provided to the patient on admission. The brochure contains
  o pictures of the hospitalists with brief biographical sketches
  o how to contact the hospitalist
  o the relationship between the hospitalist and referring physician, including how the two communicate
  o why the patient is under the care of a hospitalist instead of the patient's personal physician (i.e., advantages of the hospitalist model)
  o what the patient and family can do to maximize the chances of a good outcome from the hospital stay (e.g., follow-up with referring physician, compliance with prescribed treatments)
- The hospitalist clarifies with the patient, family, and home care provider when to contact the PCP and when to contact the hospitalist if questions arise.

- The administrative staff person contacts the hospitalist (e.g., by text message) regarding incoming questions about previously discharged patients.
- The hospitalist outlines expectations regarding daily visits, availability for family meetings, status updates, and timely discussion of test results and management decisions.
- The hospitalist uses lay terms and language that foster patients' understanding of their condition.
- The hospitalist coordinates and/or provides complete patient education regarding the plan of care upon transition from the hospital.
- The hospitalist may consider calling patients after discharge to review discharge instructions, medications, and follow-up instructions.
- The hospitalist may consider providing the patient with a copy of the discharge summary and other relevant documents at the time of discharge (often possible if stat transcription is available) or later via mail.

COMMUNICATION WITH NURSES AND OTHER HEALTHCARE STAFF

- Create a daily listing of hospitalists on duty, corresponding beeper numbers, and the patients they are following. Distribute this to all nursing units, the hospital operator, and any other party who may need to know, such as the hospitalist practice manager or rounding assistant.
- Ensure that the hospital chart clearly indicates which hospitalist is seeing the patient daily. This requires an entry in the physician orders and/or progress notes section when a change occurs in which the hospitalist is seeing the patient.
- Consider designating teams of hospitalists and label charts accordingly. Then one pager number can be assigned to each team, simplifying the mechanism of contacting the appropriate hospitalist.

- Display the hospitalist monthly schedule at nursing units and at the hospital operator switchboard.

COMMUNICATION AMONG HOSPITALISTS

- Written and concomitant verbal sign-out of patients at change of shift is most effective. Elements to consider in the handoff include
  o patient identification
  o active problems/medical history
  o active medications and allergies
  o venous access status and contingencies
  o pertinent laboratory data
  o concerns for next 18 to 24 hours
  o psychosocial status, long-term plans, and code status
- Hospitalists can consider making themselves available via beeper to other hospitalists for special questions that may arise once they leave the hospital.

Job Description for a Hospitalist Program Medical Director[1]

GENERAL DESCRIPTION

The Medical Director represents the medical leadership for the Hospitalist Program and its staff, patients, and the community. The performance of the Physician Coordinator/Medical Director sets the stage and example for all aspects of the delivery of medical services.

QUALIFICATIONS

- Licensed physician and member of Medical Staff
- Extensive training and/or experience in hospital medicine
- Career interest in hospital medicine and medical administration
- Board certification or eligibility in internal medicine
- Advanced Cardiac Life Support certification
- Long-term interest in Southwestern Vermont Health Care

ACCOUNTABLE TO

Chief Operating Officer, Chief of Staff

DUTIES AND RESPONSIBILITIES

A. Operational Management

1. Hold regular documented meetings (at least monthly) with center providers/physician extenders to discuss systems/patient flow quality, improvement in scheduling, and patient and physician relationships.
2. Participate and regularly meet at least monthly with MPD center manager and/or SVHC administration to review progress of hospitalist programs.
3. Assist in the professional development and growth of each individual provider and/or physician extenders.
4. Assist, regularly review, and annually sign off on, as approved and updated, the latest Joint Commission standard policies, procedures, and medical protocols regarding patient care.
5. In conjunction with the Chief of Staff provide guidance to hospitalist program services to include policies, personnel, services, marketing, quality assurance monitoring, and education.
6. Regularly assess center medical staff perceptions and needs of the program to ensure a harmonious working relationship, provides leadership to practitioners resulting in overall center improvement by
    a. encouraging teamwork and participation
    b. assisting in any necessary face-to-face or phone interviews, recruitment, placement, counseling, and/or termination of physicians
    c. orienting new providers and monitoring their ongoing compliance with policies and procedures
    d. coordinating provider scheduling to ensure efficiency and maximum productivity
    e. being responsible for receiving, investigating, and settling in conjunction with the Chief of Staff all grievances or questions of policy concerning and/or raised by medical providers/physician extenders

f. reviewing, investigating, managing, and reporting all complaints concerning physician staff/physician extenders arising from patients, medical staff, or administration (Appropriate complaint disposition will include reporting in writing to Chief Operating Officer and Chief of Staff.)

g. providing clinical leadership and overall supervision to all physician extenders assigned to center

h. interceding in and providing counseling, retraining, direction, and discipline to medical staff regarding contract and productivity issues

7. Regularly attend other medical staff committees, as negotiated with Chief of Staff.

8. Work closely with the Chief Operating Officer/Chief of Staff to achieve the corporation's goals for contract stability and optimal contract management.

9. Provide direct patient care in hospitalist program, 13 shifts per four-week block.

10. Provide overall medical leadership to all members associated with the practice.

11. Participate in negotiations of new center physicians/extenders relative to contracts and contract changes.

12. Assist in an efficient and expeditious operation of the practice, providing input on budgets, billing, equipment, staffing, and yearly goals and objectives.

13. Interact closely with administration to develop goals and provide ongoing assessment to achieve objectives, in keeping with hospital's strategic plan(s).

14. Work cooperatively and supportively with the center administration and physicians to ensure services are available and cost effective, meeting quality and regulatory guidelines.

15. Complete the following reports on time: Quality Assurance, Physician Interview, Evaluation, and Complaint reports.

16. Attend corporation's physician/provider retreats.

17. Conduct ongoing monitoring of compliance with hospital and center's risk management program.

18. Interact with the center/hospital medical staff and specialists to ensure appropriate and timely patient care, patient transfers, and patient referrals.
19. Interact closely with administration to develop goals and ongoing assessment of achieving objectives.
20. Work cooperatively and supportively with the heads of diagnostic and therapeutic departments to ensure availability and effective use of services and results reporting.

B. Marketing

1. Assist in the development and implementation of marketing and public relation plans.
2. Promote/ensure patient satisfaction in all areas of patient care delivery.
3. Represent center at requested community functions, presentations, and meetings/forums.

C. Quality Improvement

1. Assist with development and maintenance of continuous quality improvement programs, ensuring
   a. monitoring and supporting medical quality improvement plan and peer review processes,
   b. continuous monitoring and assurance of compliance of physician quality of care/safety programs, and
   c. completion of quarterly quality assurance/safety provider performance reviews.
2. Promote and monitor provider attendance at physician hospital organization and physician staff meetings.
3. Ensure the center achieves/passes/meets and maintains Joint Commission managed care and other accreditations.
4. Assist in development, coordination, and completion of educational programs for providers, staff, patients, and community.
5. Oversee compliance with managed care requirements, including timely and appropriate medication formulary utilization and specialist referrals.

D. Other

1. Responsible for other duties that may be defined in the bylaws of the hospital Medical Staff and/or as designated by the hospital, Chief Executive Officer, Chief of Staff, and/or their designees.

NOTE

1. Reprinted with permission from Dr. Novotny, Southwestern Vermont Health Care, Bennington, Vermont.

Sample Performance Dashboards
for a Hospitalist Program

Presented on the following pages are two sample performance dashboards. As discussed in Chapter 15, reports are often complex, voluminous, and overly detailed. Thus, it is important to select a handful of key business indicators to summarize the information. The most important performance indicators can be presented by a dashboard.

Metric	Target	Actual		Trend	Status
		Current Quarter	Previous Quarter		
Volume: Total Inpatient encounters	4,800 or higher	3,786	3,259	⇧	●
Case Mix: Medicare CMI	1.06 or higher	.098	.099	⇨	●
Patient Satisfaction: Press-Ganey "Physician Communication" score	85th percentile or higher	64%	58%	⇧	●
Length of Stay: Medicare LOS for inpatient admissions with medicine DRGs	4.2 or lower	4.1	4.8	⇧	●
Hospital Cost: Average cost per discharge	$3,650 or lower	3,827	3,692	⇨	●
Ancillary Utility: Pharmacy unit doses per discharge	50 or lower	46	49	⇨	●
Productivity: wRVUs per FTE	900	943	868	⇧	●
Provider Satisfaction: "Overall Satisfaction" score on survey instrument	4.0 or higher (on 5-point scale)	3.8	2.8	⇧	●
Mortality: Full-code patients expiring outside the ICU	Zero	0	2	⇧	●
Readmission Rate: Percent of patients readmitted within 72 hours of same dx	3% or lower	2.8%	2.5%	⇨	●

Source: Reprinted with permission from Leslie Flores, Nelson/Flores Associates, LLC.

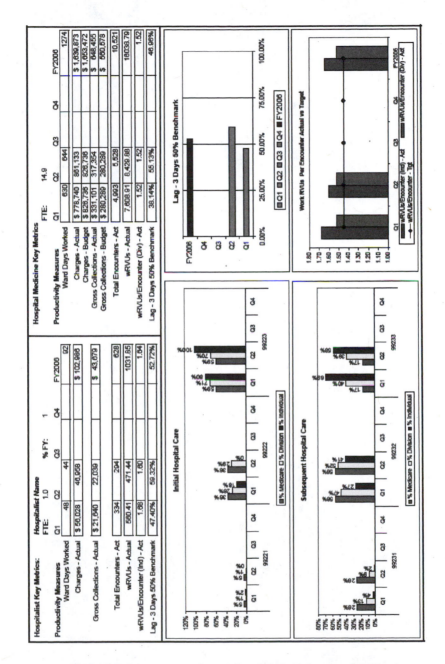

Source: Reprinted with permission from Edward Fink, University of California, San Diego.

Index

A

Academic institutions, 9, 10, 11–12; compensation and, 160; employment model and, 54, 56; formal education and, 40; pediatric hospitalist programs and, 214, 215, 216, 220; scheduling and, 142

ACGME (Accreditation Council for Graduate Medical Education), 12, 24, 41

Administrative support staff, 130–31

Ambulatory Pediatric Association Hospital Medicine Special Interest Group, 219

American Academy of Pediatrics, 219

American Board of Internal Medicine, 4

American Pediatric Association, 219

Antikickback statute, 78, 80, 88

Antitrust law, 88

Autonomy/control, 96

Availability. See 24/7 coverage

B

Benefits provided by hospitalists, 17–46; education and, 39–44; extraordinary availability and, 32–34; medical staffs and, 20–26; patient safety/quality of care and, 44–46; physicians' offices and, 26–31; resource utilization and, 34–37; throughput/patient flow and, 37–39; unassigned patients and, 18–20; *See also* Value added by hospitalists

Billing, 201–7; avoiding failure and, 72; incentive-based compensation and, 83; information systems and, 196, 198; medical directors and, 180–81; PAs/NPs and, 104, 105; pediatric hospitalist programs and, 216–18; practice operations and, 205–7; production-based incentives and, 202–3; rounding assistants and, 109; service, 201, 203–5; staffing and, 126, 131; success and, 69–70

Brochures, 70, 115, 117

Burnout, 93–95; night coverage and, 140, 152; scheduling and, 138, 139, 142, 143

C

Care/case managers, 102, 108, 131

Career counseling, 41

Career satisfaction, 93–100, 140, 151

Career Satisfaction Task Force, 95

Case-rate compensation, 168

Centers for Medicare & Medicaid Services. See CMS

Characteristics of hospitalists, 1–3

Charge capture, 196, 198, 205

Charges/collections, benchmarks on hospitalist, 54

Children's Hospital Boston, 42

Clinical care coordinators. See Care/case managers

Clinical metrics, 186–87

Clinical responsibilities: contracts and, 82, 86–87; of medical directors, 178–79; of PAs/NPs, 104

CMS (Centers for Medicare and Medicaid Services), 160, 165, 216

Coding, 217–18; avoiding failure and, 72; billing and, 203–4; compensation and, 164; information systems and, 196; pediatric hospitalist programs and, 211, 216–17; success and, 69; undercoding, 202

Cogent, 15

Collections, 202–3

Communication, 111–18; information systems and, 192; medical directors and, 181; multispecialty/primary care medical groups organizational model and, 13; pediatric hospitalist programs and, 220; success and, 70

Community/environment, 96

Compensation, 157–73; amount of, 159–61; benefits compensation/benchmarks, 56–57; committee, 183; employment contracts and, 83, 84; medical directors and, 176–77; methods of, 162–70; models, 54, 203, 204; night coverage and, 148, 149–50; pediatric hospitalist programs and, 215–17; productivity and, 160, 161; professional services contracts and,

87–88; recruitment and, 68; sources of revenue and, 158; special situations, 171–72; See also Incentive-based compensation

Compensation and Productivity Survey, 2005-2006, 123

Compliance, 24

Consolidated Omnibus Budget Reconciliation Act, 18

Continuity, 134, 139; pediatric hospitalist programs and, 214; scheduling and, 143

Contracts: employment, 81–86; professional services, 86–89

Core competencies in hospital medicine, 4, 5

Core Competencies in Hospital Medicine: A Framework for Curriculum Development, 4

Cost per stay/case, 36, 77; incentive-based compensation and, 83; professional services contracts and, 87; reducing, 57; Stark law and, 80

Courtesy admissions, 73

Coverage requirements. See 24/7 coverage

Covered services, 86

CPOE systems, 24, 25, 129

CPT (Current Procedural Terminology), 160, 217

Credentialing, 83

D

Daily census, 125–27; information systems and, 194–96; scheduling and, 135

Dashboard, 188–89

Decision/organizational control, 96

Disaster planning, 24

Discharge planning: communication and, 70, 115; pediatric hospitalist programs and, 212; professional services contracts and, 87; throughput and, 38; unassigned patients and, 19

Documentation, 202

E

EDs (emergency departments): extraordinary availability of hospitalists and, 32; how hospitalists provide benefits to, 28–29, 31; pediatric hospitalist programs and, 210, 213; professional services contracts and, 87; throughput and, 38; unassigned patients and, 18

Education, 6, 39–44

eHealth Initiative, 24

Electronic health records, 24

EmCare, 15

Emergency departments. See EDs

Employment contracts, 81–86

Employment model, 54, 56

EMTALA (Emergency Medical Treatment and Labor Act), 18

Ethics in Patient Referrals Act. See Stark law

Exclusivity clauses, 88, 89

Expenses, projected, 56–57

Expertise of hospitalists, 1, 2, 3–4

F

Failure, avoiding, 70–75

Federal Office of the National Coordinator for Health Information Technology, 24

Financial issues: avoiding failure and financial support, 74–75; financial benefits, 57–60; information systems and, 192; value added by hospitalists and, 6

Fixed/variable salary, 164–67

Formal education, 40–41

FTE (full-time equivalent), 84; compensation and, 171; medical directors and, 182; night coverage and, 150, 151; pediatric hospitalist programs and, 214; staffing and, 121–24, 126–27

G

Gainsharing, 78, 80–81, 83

H

Handoffs, 112, 134, 136

Health Insurance Portability and Accountability Act of 1996, 24

Hospitals/hospital-owned corporations, 9–11

I

Incentive-based compensation, 157, 166; employment contracts and, 83; organizational models and, 11; pediatric hospitalist programs and, 216–17; professional services contracts and, 87; sample approaches to, 170; success and, 64–65; See also Production-based incentives

Independent contractors, 82, 85, 86

Informal education, 40, 43

Information systems, 24, 191–98; basic, 192–97; pediatric hospitalist programs and, 216; sophisticated, 197–98

Institute of Medicine, 24

Intensive care, 38; *See also* NICU; PICU

IPC-The Hospitalist Co., 15

J

Jeopardy, doctors on, 67

Job-fit questionnaire, 97

Joint Commission, 24, 65, 112, 186

K

Kaiser Permanente, 213

L

Leadership: avoiding failure and, 71; career satisfaction and principles of, 99; communication and, 116–18; compensation and, 171; council, 183; medical directors and, 175, 177, 180; physician, 21–22, 25; success and, 64

Leapfrog Group, 24, 38

Legal issues, 77–81, 88; methods of compensation and, 162; PAs/NPs and, 105; See also Contracts

Length of stay. *See* LOS

Local hospitalist-only groups, 9–10, 13–14; employment model and, 54

Log books, 192–94

LOS (length of stay), 77, 78; billing and, 205; compensation and, 83, 168; extraordinary availability of hospitalists and, 33; gainsharing and, 81; information systems and, 196; pediatric hospitalist programs and, 211–12, 214; performance measurement and, 185, 186, 187; professional services contracts and, 87; reducing, 36–37, 38, 57; Stark law and, 80; workloads and, 96

Lost charges, 202

M

Malpractice insurance, 85

Managed care organization. See MCO

Management companies. *See* Multistate hospitalist-only group/management companies

Managing relationships, 176

Markle Foundation, 24

Mayo Clinic study, 28

MCO (managed care organization), 87, 88

Medicaid: pediatric hospitalist programs and, 211; Stark law and, 78; unassigned patients and, 19

Medical directors, 175–84; assistant, 181; compensation and, 157; hiring, 176–77; managing relationships and, 176; responsibilities of, 177–81; revenue and, 201; successful positioning for, 181–84

Medical staffs, 20–26

Medicare, 55, 56, 78

MGMA (Medical Group Management Association), 123, 159

Mitretek Systems, 21

Modern Healthcare, 159

Moffitt-Long Hospital, 42

Moonlighting, 82–83, 127, 141, 216

Mount Zion Hospital, 42

Multispecialty/primary care medical groups, 9, 12–13; employment model and, 54, 56; overhead and, 73

Multistate hospitalist-only group/management companies, 9, 10, 14–15, 197; employment model and, 54; largest, 15

N

National Institute for Children's Healthcare Quality, 219

National Patient Safety Goals, 112

NICU (neonatal intensive care unit), 210, 214, 217

Night coverage, 32, 145–54; arrangements for, 146–49; benefits of, 152; compensation and, 149–50, 157, 171; decision framework for, 148; increasing productivity of, 152–54; pediatric hospitalist programs and, 214, 215; practice economics related to, 150–52; scheduling and, 139–41, 146; staffing and, 130; success and, 65–66

Nocturnists, 66, 147, 151, 152, 153, 154

Nonclinical responsibilities, 25; contracts and, 82; of medical directors, 179–81; staffing and, 128, 129

Norwalk Hospital, Connecticut, 42

NPs (nurse practitioners), 102–8; pediatric hospitalist programs and, 218; staffing and, 130

Nurses, 24, 131, 152, 154, 210

O

Observation codes, 218

OIG (Office of Inspector General), 78, 80

On-call physicians, 32, 145, 147, 148, 151, 154; scheduling and, 137; unassigned patients and, 18–19
Operational metrics, 186–87
Oregon Health and Science University, 42
Organizational models, 9–15
Overhead, 72–73, 158
Oversight committee, 71, 183

P

Partnership tracks, 85–86
PAs (physician assistants), 24, 102–8, 130, 218
Patients, communication with, 114–16, 117
Patient satisfaction, 23
Patient volume, 66–67
Pay for performance. *See* P4P
P4P (pay for performance), 44, 55–56
PCPs (primary care physicians), 26–31; information systems and, 197; moonlighting and, 127; night coverage and, 153–54; perception of hospitalists by, 30; staffing and, 122
Pediatric hospitalist programs, 209–21; billing/coding, 217–18; compensation/incentives, 215–17; economics of, 211–14; NPs/PAs and, 218; organizational resources for, 218–19; other considerations for, 220; scheduling/staffing, 214–15; what they do, 210–11
Pediatric Hospital Medicine listserv, 219
Pediatric intensive care unit. See PICU
Performance measurement, 68–69, 185–90
Performance reporting, 192
Perioperative consults, 123
Physical environment control, 96
Physician assistants. See PAs
Physician Compensation and Production Survey, 123
Physician perceptions of hospitalists, 30
Physician Quality Reporting Initiative, 56
Physicians, communication with referring, 112–14, 115–16, 117
Physician schedules, 65–66
PICU (pediatric intensive care unit), 210, 213, 214, 217
Political support, 183–84
Practice guidelines, 23, 25, 36, 129
Practice managers, 182–83
Primary care physicians. See PCPs

PrimeDoc, 15

Production-based incentives, 69, 72, 166, 167–71, 201, 202–3, 204; pediatric
    hospitalist programs and, 216; success and, 65

Productivity and Compensation Survey, 78

Professional-fee revenues, 51–52, 53, 75, 77, 158

Professional liability insurance, 85, 88

Professional services contracts, 86–89

Q

QI (Quality improvement), 23

Quality incentives, 65, 166, 167, 170

Quality of care: extraordinary availability of hospitalists and, 33; improving,
    44–46; incentive-based compensation and, 83; night coverage and, 140,
    152; pediatric hospitalist programs and, 213; value added by hospitalists
    and, 6

Quality of Health Care in America (Committee of the Institute of Medicine), 44

R

Recruitment, 129; avoiding failure and, 71; compensation and, 157, 163; medical
    directors and, 176, 177, 181, 182; night coverage and, 152; pediatric hospi-
    talist programs and, 217, 220; scheduling and, 143; success and, 67–68

Referrals, staffing and, 122, 123

Relative value units (RVUs), 160

Renewability, of contracts, 82

Reporting requirements, 87

Reports: billing service, 204; performance measurement and, 188

Residency programs, 41; pediatric hospitalist programs and, 220; recruitment
    and, 68

Resource control, 96

Resource utilization, 34–37

Restrictive covenants, 88, 89

Retention. *See* Career satisfaction

Return on investment. See ROI

Revenues, 53–56, 158

Reward/recognition, 96

ROI (return on investment), 51–60; financial benefits and, 57–60; pediatric
    hospitalist programs and, 211, 218; performance measurement and, 189;
    projected expenses and, 56–57; projected revenues and, 53–56

Rounding assistants, 102, 108–9, 131

S

Safety, patient, 23–24; improving, 44–46; value added by hospitalists and, 6

Scheduling, 133–43; career satisfaction and, 96; checklist for evaluating, 135; elements of, 134, 136–41; employment contracts and, 83–85; information systems and, 192; mapping, 141–42; medical directors and, 181, 182; pediatric hospitalist programs and, 214–15; physicians and, 65–66; production-based compensation and, 169; 7-on/7off, 142–43; staffing and, 128–29; See *also* Night coverage

Senior population, 37

7-on/7-off scheduling, 142–43

Shifts, 137, 138, 142, 143, 145; See *also* Night coverage

Software vendors, 197

Staffing, 121–31; estimating FTE requirements and, 121–24; medical directors and, 181; models, 24; nonphysician, 101–9, 130–31; other approaches to estimating requirements for, 125–27; pediatric hospitalist programs and, 214–15; practice attributes and increasing/decreasing FTE requirements, 127–30; production-based compensation and, 168, 169; scheduling and, 134, 137

Stark law, 78–80, 82, 83, 87–88

Steering committee, 183

Straight/fixed salary, 163–64

Success, achieving, 63–70

Surgeons, 27–28, 31, 210

Surgical comanagement, 28, 38, 74

Sweeps clauses, 88, 89

T

Tail coverage, 85

Task control, 96

TeamHealth, 15

Term, of contracts, 82

Termination, of contracts, 82

Throughput, 6, 28–29, 37–39

To Err Is Human: Building a Safer Health System, 44

Transparency, 44

24/7 coverage, 6, 32–34, 125, 134, 214; See *also* Night coverage

U

Unassigned patients, 18–20; avoiding failure and, 74; staffing and, 122–23
Undercoding, 202
University of California, San Francisco, 59
University of Chicago, 42
Utilization management, 88
Utilization review, 23, 25, 87, 88, 129

V

Value added by hospitalists, 2, 4–6; See *also* Benefits provided by hospitalists
Volunteering, 21

W

Weekend work, 141
"Winterist" physicians, 215
Workloads: avoiding failure and, 74; career satisfaction and, 96; compensation and, 163; medical directors and, 181; pediatric hospitalist programs and, 214, 215; scheduling and, 137, 138, 139; staffing and, 126–27, 128–29, 130
Work relative value units (wRVUs), 65; billing and, 205, 206; compensation and, 160, 165, 168, 204; production-based incentives and, 203; staffing and, 122

About the Authors

Joseph A. Miller is senior vice president for the Society of Hospital Medicine (SHM). In this role, Mr. Miller oversees SHM's membership/marketing functions, data management/web services, and business operations. In addition, he coordinates SHM's biannual Productivity and Compensation Survey, staffs the SHM Benchmarks Committee and Career Satisfaction Task Force, and is course director for SHM's Practice Management Pre-Course. Mr. Miller does part-time hospitalist consulting with Dr. Winthrop Whitcomb, with whom he cofounded Northeast Hospitalist Consulting. He has more than 30 years of management, consulting, and market research experience with provider organizations, health plans, academic institutions, and vendors.

John Nelson, M.D., FACP, is one of the founders of the hospitalist movement and has been a practicing hospitalist since 1988. He is a hospitalist and the hospitalist program's medical director at Overlake Hospital in Bellevue, Washington. Since 1994, he has been working with institutions around the United States to start new hospitalist practices or to improve existing ones. He is the founder of Nelson/Flores Associates, a consulting firm that provides guidance for hospitalist practices. Dr. Nelson serves on the faculty for the Hospitalist Practice Management Course sponsored by SHM. He, along with Dr. Winthrop Whitcomb, cofounded SHM and has served as its past president.

Winthrop F. Whitcomb, M.D., has been a practicing hospitalist since 1994 at Mercy Medical Center in Springfield, Massachusetts. From 1994 through 2004, he served as director of the Mercy Inpatient Medicine Service, America's first and most widely emulated program with 24/7 on-site hospitalist staffing. Since cofounding SHM in 1996, he has been widely recognized as a principal leader of the U.S. hospitalist movement and the field of hospital medicine. Currently, Dr. Whitcomb serves as director of performance improvement at Mercy Medical Center and as director of hospitalist services for Catholic Health East, a 42-hospital system in the eastern United States. He is assistant professor of medicine at the University of Massachusetts Medical School. He has provided consultation to hospitalist programs throughout the United States since 1996.

ABOUT THE CONTRIBUTORS

David L. Bernd, FACHE, is chief executive officer of Sentara Healthcare, an integrated health system with net revenues of $2.5 billion. Sentara, a not-for-profit healthcare provider in southeastern Virginia and northeastern North Carolina, is composed of seven acute care hospitals, health plans with 340,000 covered lives, and 300 physician medical groups. Sentara was ranked the number one integrated healthcare network in the United States in 2001 by *Modern Healthcare* magazine, and it is the only healthcare system to be named in the top 10 for the past nine years. Most recently, Mr. Bernd, was appointed by the Secretary of Commerce to serve as a member of the Measuring Innovation in the 21st Century Economy Advisory Committee of the Department of Commerce. In 2004, he served as chairman of the American Hospital Association Board of Trustees, making him the top elected official of the largest hospital and health system association in the United States. In addition, he is a Fellow of the American College of Healthcare Executives (ACHE). Mr. Bernd was the 1984 recipient of the American College of Hospital Administrators's (now ACHE) Robert S. Hudgens National Young

Hospital Administrator of the Year Award. Mr. Bernd contributed the Foreword to this book.

Leslie Flores is an experienced healthcare executive and consultant. She has held a variety of executive-level positions in Southern California hospitals, with responsibility for clinical and support services as well as for staff functions in strategic planning and business development, managed care, community benefit planning, and physician recruitment and practice development. Since 1999, Ms. Flores has been providing management consulting, training, and leadership development services for hospitals, physician groups, and other healthcare organizations. Currently, she is a partner at Nelson/Flores Associates, LLC, a consulting practice that specializes in building successful new hospital medicine programs and enhancing the effectiveness and value of existing programs. Ms. Flores contributed Chapter 15 to this book.

Jack M. Percelay, M.D., M.P.H., FAAP, is a national leader in the pediatric hospital medicine movement. He has more than 17 years of experience as a pediatric hospitalist in a wide variety of community hospital settings, including the pediatric ward, pediatric intensive care unit (ICU), neonatal ICU, and emergency department. He has led single and multisite hospitalist practices and regularly speaks, writes, and consults on pediatric hospital medicine systems of care. Dr. Percelay has coauthored national guidelines for pediatric hospital medicine programs and serves on several national groups that examine quality measures and standards for pediatric care. He is a charter member of SHM and currently serves as secretary and pediatric representative on the SHM board. Dr. Percelay contributed Chapter 18 to this book.

The Society of Hospital Medicine is the premier medical society representing hospitalists, physicians whose primary focus is the care of hospitalized patients. For more information about SHM, visit www.hospitalmedicine.org.